How To Live To 100
(and enjoy it!)

By Chris Cawood
Magnolia Hill Press
Kingston, Tennessee

Book Number:_____/2000

_____

Author Autograph

Printed in the United States of America

Library of Congress Catalog Card Number 96-94049

ISBN 0-9642231-1-2

Dedication

I dedicate this book to the memory of my two long-lived grandmothers, Belle Crutchfield Hatmaker Trotter, 1880-1974; and Lillie Jones Cawood Reed, 1899-1994, who endured through bad times and good with indomitable determination and spry spirits, always looking to the future.

"The days of our years are threescore years and ten; and if by reason of strength they be fourscore years; yet is their strength labor and sorrow; for it is soon cut off, and we fly away . . . .

"So teach us to number our days: that we may apply our hearts unto wisdom."—Psalms 90: 10 & 12

"Honor thy father and thy mother: that thy days may be long upon the land which the Lord thy God giveth thee."—Exodus 20: 12.

Introduction

J ust ordinary men and women. This is how those whose stories follow described themselves.

"Why are you here? Why do you want to talk with me? I have never done anything of note." They just lived—and lived, and lived.

When these men and women were born in the late 1880s and through the mid-1890s, the average life expectancy for men and women combined was **45 years**. These extraordinary people have exceeded that expectancy by more than double. What enabled them to do it? And are there lessons in their stories for us?

These men and women have seen the changes of a century. All but two are native Tennesseans. The state was born in 1796. They were born about a hundred years later. And as I finish this book in 1996—the Bicentennial year—these Tennessee Treasures are half as old as the state.

At the time of their births, there were no radios, no automobiles, no airplanes, no cellophane, no zippers, no stainless steel, no sulfa drugs, no Social Security, and no minimum wage. There were just forty-four states, and women couldn't vote.

On a personal level, transportation was actually in the horse and buggy age. Long trips were made by train, or else as adventurous pilgrimages on horses or behind them. Roads were dirt in the country and often in the towns. Cars and planes would arrive during their lifetimes, but at birth it was the train or the river.

There were a few electric lights strung in the large towns, and the telephone was making its way to the big cities. But in the country there was none of that.

They lived through several wars, the Great Depression, and the influenza epidemic of 1918-19 that literally decimated the population in parts of the country.

Now, from behind clouded eyes, they can still see the world of their youth if they're asked. They don't live in the past, but they will visit it if invited. Sometimes they have to think hard to remember what it was like. But when they pull the nuggets of the past through the fire of remembrance, they are worth considering. They are, as we all are, people of the present looking to the future.

They still do what they always did—only slower and with more effort.

Their sight is dimmed, their hearing dulled, and their skin wrinkled and leathered, but their spirits thrive, encased within clay cocoons. When they think back, a smile grows, a glint shines through their eyes, or a hand gestures as if it were just yesterday.

I imagine them, as they hesitate to answer a question, rewinding the ragged movie film of their minds and seeing the old house, the school, the car, or the father or mother I'm asking about. I want the whole reel, but they give me only glimpses—snapshots of yesterday.

An uncle lost a foot in the Civil War. "His wooden foot is over in the museum at Norris." "My folks kept bee hives in the attic." "I drove a blind horse to my brother's wedding and got the wagon stuck in a deep mud hole." "My father bought me a piano. Oh, how I loved to play, and my father loved to listen." "I told the preacher to come back in the summer so I could be baptized for real in the river."

There are now estimated to be 52,000 centenarians in

the United States. The U.S. Census Bureau projects that by the year 2040 there will be 1.3 million Americans 100 years or older. Those *Baby Boomers* who are now beginning to turn fifty and who make up the largest segment of our population will be among that group.

"The only person who wants to live to 100 is the person who is 99," one centenarian said. That is translated to mean that we don't necessarily look forward to getting *old* but we do look forward to getting *older* when we consider the alternative.

I am not a sociologist, psychologist, or gerontologist. My conclusions in chapters that are interspersed in this book are based on observations of the ones I interviewed. The individuals were not part of *case studies* as such. I just talked with them and recorded their responses and my notes. I didn't ask them how they lived to be a hundred. I doubt if they knew.

Interviews and research for the book began in 1993 and continued through the early part of 1996. Many of the ones that grace these pages have now passed on, but their stories are told because I think they are important. One whom I interviewed at ninety-seven years of age died shortly before reaching one hundred. His story is included.

This is not pure history nor social history. These are stories of ordinary people who made the state what it is. They speak to us through a hundred years of experience, but they don't try to lecture us—they know it wouldn't work. Some of their memories include fathers, mothers, uncles, and grandparents whose lives take us back to the early to mid 1800s.

My thanks is to them and their children who helped me arrange to talk with them. May we learn from their lives and enjoy their stories.

Chris Cawood—Kingston, Tennessee, February, 1996.

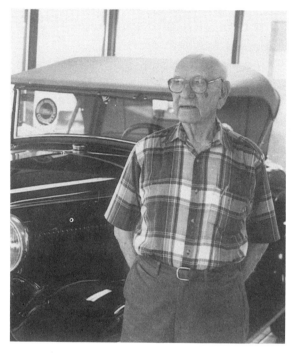

William Franklin Jarnagin
Grainger County—December 8,1894

On an early June morning, I drove to Rutledge, which straddles Highway 11W and is the county seat of Grainger. About a half hour out of Knoxville on the left is the relatively new home of Jarnagin Ford. Down the road a bit is a Hardee's, and along the way are signs advertising the most famous tomatoes in East Tennessee.

This is rural East Tennessee where lush green grass grows on fields that slope from ridge to ridge. The famous tomatoes mature in rich brown dirt that is watered this morning by a light rain. Clouds roll in like steel wool above a green carpet. From time to time an abandoned old farmhouse is visible from the newly-paved highway. With just a little imagination, I am transported back over the years to a time when roads were dirt and trains were the means of long rides to Knoxville or Middlesboro, Kentucky.

When I arrive, Bill Jarnagin sits in the showroom talking with his ninety-three-year-old brother, a younger cousin, and his grandson who now runs the family business. He gets up and shakes my hand with a firm grip that would be expected in a man thirty years younger. Near six feet in height, he walks to a small office off the showroom floor and sits behind a desk heaped with mementos.

Just a few miles south lies the site of his birth, a family farm that covered many acres when he was born but has now shrunken in size. Jarnagins have been in that part of Grainger County for at least a hundred fifty years, maybe more.

Bill believes his ancestors were English, and they came to America in the 1700s. "They followed the rivers into the area." In the early to mid-1800s they walked in from Virginia or North Carolina and settled in this rustic valley, through which went the main road from Washington to the west.

By the time of the Civil War, the family had several hundred acres in farm land and, like the majority of East Tennesseans, were pro-Union.

A small skirmish of the Civil War was fought on their land with a cannon shell splitting a Catawba tree that survived and is a testament to that encounter to this day.

"My father was about ten years old when they shot the top out of that tree. He told me the story many times. 'Boy, get down in the cellar and stay there,' his father told him."

Bill Jarnagin, when I talked with him in June 1995, was still coming to work every day—five and a half days a week. He had moved a son and his wife into his house where they looked after each other.

"I get here about seven-thirty and leave around five-thirty."

He thought back and laughed. "I even came in this past Memorial Day. I forgot we weren't open until I got here and nobody else came in. I had me a cup of coffee and went back home."

Born the fourth of nine children of William A. Jarnagin and Launa McCarty Jarnagin, Bill remembers his father as a farmer, blacksmith, and horse breeder. Hard work as a youth consisted of working the bellows for his father's blacksmithing fire.

"Every rainy day I'd have to pump them old bellows. They were getting old. You never seen none I don't guess. You had a handle on them, and you had to pump them up and down."

School amounted to close to a hundred students being shepherded by one teacher at Red House and then a bit later at Little Valley. Red House was just a mile from his home, and he and his brothers and sisters walked the wagon road in good weather or along the railroad track when the road was muddy.

With too many students at Red House, the school marm insisted that the Jarnagins and Renfros go to Little Valley. The next year she was transferred to Little Valley and insisted that they go back to Red House.

"I just don't think she wanted to take care of a hundred of us."

As we talked more in his little office, he showed me the just-framed certificates and commendations he received the past December on his hundredth birthday. For seventy-nine years he has been involved in a Ford dealership. He'd met members of the Ford family at different functions over the years. It was a lot different in 1916 when he first helped a cousin go into business.

Looking back on it now, it was rather ironic that the first Fords shipped to the Jarnagin dealership in Rutledge arrived by train. The autos would eventually just about put the passenger trains out of business.

"They took them to Bean Station. I had to go up there and assemble them."

Assemble them?

"Yeah, they came unassembled. We had to build a machine to lift them out of the boxcars and then put them together.

"I helped carry the first chassis out. Then we pulled the motor out and the wheels. Ford Motor has forgotten they shipped them that way."

From his cousin, John R. Jarnagin, Bill later received an interest in the dealership, which is now the oldest continuous active Ford dealership in the country.

Before the dealership, Bill Jarnagin worked as a mechanic in Knoxville on Vine Street near the intersection of Depot and Central. He roomed in a boarding house.

When the United States entered World War I, he was the right age to go. But he had a special talent as an auto mechanic. There was an Automobile Division in Knoxville. He joined up, but the war was over in three and a half months.

"That's as far as I got. Knoxville. I didn't have to carry a gun. My job was training." He thinks back and chuckles at the idea of spending his part of the experience of World War I in Knoxville.

After the war, it was back to the Fords where a Model T sold for $425.

He married Jenny Byerly in 1919, and they had three children. Jenny and a daughter both died of cancer while a son was killed in an automobile accident.

LIGHTS TO RUTLEDGE

Before TVA, Bill Jarnagin was a pioneer of sorts in bringing electricity to Rutledge—at least the houses that were near the dealership.

"We needed some electric power for our building so we got the Delco people out here to engineer us a system. They thought a three kilowatt generator would be enough. I didn't know what a kilowatt was but found out pretty soon that we needed more.

"We had three T Model Ford tractors that we couldn't sell. So, I ordered a ten kilowatt generator, bolted it to the floor, and hooked up the tractor engines to run it. We ran the exhaust out the back wall.

"Had more electricity than we could use. We put poles and wires up and ran electricity to forty or fifty nearby houses and businesses. We charged a $2.50 flat rate until some started to steal the power. Then we had to buy meters.

"We burned out those tractor engines, burst engine blocks, and popped out lights by overpowering them. I got tired of trying to keep it running and sold out to Bettis Electric Company over in Morristown."

The Depression hit car dealerships hard. Few people had money for anything other than the bare necessities. Even years before the stock market crash of 1929, car sales began to slump. From the $425 for a Model T in 1917, Henry Ford had to give special incentives and lower the price by $50 and $100 to keep people coming in.

"Around 1923, if you hand $388.10, I could put you into a touring car."

With the emergence of the automobile, big hotels that catered to the railroad traffic began to flounder. Bill's cousin, John R. Jarnagin, owned a big hotel at Tate Springs. As the automobile business went up, his hotel business went down. Fortunately, he had an interest in each.

When John R. died in 1944, Bill then became partners with his cousin's wife. Fire destroyed the business in 1957, and he had to move the location—but he never gave up. He moved, rebuilt the business, and survived to where it is the oldest in the Ford family.

After the Civil War, his family remained Republicans. Now, a grandson works and lives at the Governor's Mansion in Nashville as one of the personal guards to the Governor after over eighteen years as a Tennessee State Trooper. The other grandson runs the Ford business.

Bill walked outside with me for a picture and showed

me the parking lot where over two thousand gathered for his 100th Birthday Party.

"I'm a Baptist, but I visit around a lot at different churches. So many came to my party that I like to go and visit with them."

Bill Jarnagin is illustrative of the turn-of-the-century entrepreneur who worked hard and took risks in a new industry that was to change the face of the country.

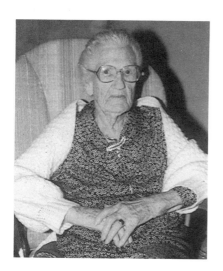
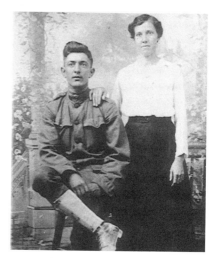

Sophia Dodson Hale
Cumberland County—October 16, 1890

Quilting and religion. Both played important and pivotal roles in the life of Sophia Dodson Hale. Born in the Cumberland County community of Winesap, she moved to neighboring White County with her family at age five and spent the rest of her life in a rural farm setting. The Dodsons were from White County and only sojourned a few years in Cumberland.

Like Bill Jarnagin's ancestors, Sophia Dodson's came to Grainger County in the late 1700s or early 1800s from

Grayson County, Virginia, but moved on to Cumberland and White Counties. There they settled along the picturesque Caney Fork River.

Longevity ran in the family. A great-great grandfather is said to have lived to be 114. Her mother lived to 86 and her father to one month short of 95.

Sophia was the sixth of twelve children born to Harvey Mansfield Dodson and Betty Ann McCormick Dodson. Ten lived to maturity—five boys and five girls. On a cool February morning when I visited with Sophia Dodson Hale, only she and a 94-year-old sister remained.

Her father's brother fought in the Civil War, but there was no talk of it around the house—at least in the presence of the children. Wars were things to be forgotten rather than re-membered. Life consisted of births, marriages, quiltings, and finding room for a dozen people in a log house.

Life was considerably different in rural Tennessee in the 1890s and early 1900s than it is now, although Sophia and the other centenarians I talked with seemed to move with relative ease from one century's lack of conveniences to the other's myriad of gadgets.

With no electricity, no cars, no bridges, and no tele-phones, people were more dependent on each other. Neighbors were not just people who lived next door or down the road but were ones who could be relied on during times of need.

Families, too, were different. They were larger and more joined by necessity at the homeplace.

"We didn't have too big a house. Old time houses were built with just a log room and then a side room for kitchens and upstairs. We had two big log rooms and a hall between them. Then we would build on extra as it was needed.

"My daddy built on an extra two rooms to our house and a big long front porch. We had a downstairs, upstairs, and a cellar. The cellar was just a dug out place to put our canned fruit and potatoes."

The Caney Fork River, although providing water for

cattle and watering rich bottom land, proved to be an obstacle also. Now, between Smithville and Nashville, Interstate 40 easily traverses the river four times as it snakes its way around the low ridges and sandy shoals. A driver hardly notices the bridges and takes them for granted.

"We didn't have no bridges then. We had dirt roads, and we forded the river on horse back or in wagons. The nearest bridge was way down. If the water was up, we'd have to go through Van Buren County to get to Sparta."

If they didn't want to take a horse or wagon across the river, there was a neighbor's boat that was used as a ferry for people.

"We just had small boats to cross. Up the river a way, there was a family who lived on each side of the river. When they'd holler over to the other side that someone needed to cross the river, the people on the other side would bring the boat across.

"There was no charge for it. That's the way they'd cross the river. Just had one boat. Sometimes it would be on one side and sometimes on the other."

The farm was self-sufficient in many ways, and few things had to be bought.

"My daddy would raise cattle, hogs, sheep, sweet potatoes, and Irish potatoes. We'd keep the potatoes by hoeing them up, putting them in a pile, and putting dirt and hay over them. They'd stay all winter.

"We mainly just had to buy salt, sugar, and soda. We raised about everything else. We'd grind our wheat at a rolling mill in Sparta, and my dad would put it in a swinging rack upstairs where the mice couldn't get to it.

"We had sheep and wool. They'd card the wool at the factory, and he'd bring it home in rolls. My mother would do the spinning. She would knit our stockings and made woolen underwear."

With ten children and an extended family all about, everyone was expected to do his or her part on the farm.

"I'd do about everything there was to do. I'd mind the babies and work in the garden. I didn't like to mind the babies. I'd rather work in the garden. I'd milk cows. We boiled our clothes in an old black pot and washed them on a scrub board."

Quilted A Husband

In rural White County, as in many places in Tennessee and the South, the social life in the early part of this century revolved around church and quiltings. The making of a quilt by a group of women at a time of celebration—such as a birthday party—served the purpose of fulfilling a utilitarian need while allowing for merriment and celebration at the same time. In a deeply religious community, the party then could be justified as not totally frivolous or tending toward the Devil's excess.

On February 15, 1913, Sophia Dodson was invited to attend a birthday party and quilting honoring a neighbor boy who was turning from adolescence into manhood at age twenty-one.

"He was twenty-one, and his mother and daddy gave him a quilting. I happened to be on Lost Creek at my brother's store up there, and I was invited to the quilting. He said that day that the best quilter would be his wife.

"All of us women just worked on one quilt. He and some of the other boys went to the store and got some chewing gum and candy. When they came back, they threw the candy around and punched the quilt, just acting crazy. Trying to get the girls' attention, I guess.

"We went together for a year and got married on his twenty-second birthday."

"Were you the best quilter there?" I asked.

"Well, I wouldn't say I was."

"At least he picked you."

"I guess I was good enough," she said and smiled. I

could almost see her going back over those decades in her mind.

"Did you think he was quite a catch?"

"Oh, he was a poor man, but he was a good husband, and we always had a happy life."

What she just said proved true with most of the centenarians who talked with me. During those times of a hundred years or so ago in rural Tennessee, wealth in the form of money or gold never appeared to be a goal. Wealth was measured by these people in the lives they lived and their relations with family and friends.

"Did he have a farm?" I asked.

"No. He had nothing. He went into the Army in 1917 and came out in 1920. He was in the trenches when the armistice was signed."

Sophia's husband being in the Army led to two of her three trips outside Tennessee.

"Have you traveled very much?"

"No, not much. I went twice to South Carolina when my husband was in the Army to visit him before he went overseas. Then I lived in Maryland for three years with my daughter."

"What about California or Florida? Ever gone there?"

She smiled slightly as though to humor her interrogator. "No, I never have been nowhere."

But looking out the window, I knew she had been just where she wanted to be. The now brown grass of winter waved gently in a slight breeze between her house and the road where a car might pass every five minutes. Beyond lay the river, and beyond that the undulating ridges of this edge of the Cumberland Plateau.

Methodist With A Memory

Back in the 1890s and early 1900s, television, radio, and the wide use of electricity were mere glimmers of inventive thought in minds far away from White County, Tennessee. There was no Oprah, televised baseball, or even the Grand Ole Opry. Entertainment came where you could find it—usually mixed with something uplifting or inspiring.

Religion met the spiritual needs of the rural, agrarian society, but it also provided respite from labor when it was time for the summer revival. Sophia Dodson was brought up a Methodist, and she remembered those meetings of long ago.

"Spiritually, our churches are just a performed worship so much more than when I was growing up. We'd use to have revivals, and they'd be big professions. People would fast and pray. Now, it's just a feast.

"They'd go to the mourners' bench and then down to the river to be baptized. We'd sing 'Shall We Gather At The River.' They were really serious.

"Those meetings would last for two weeks or at least ten days. Sometimes we'd have a service in the day as well as at night."

She paused and thought back to the time of her childhood and the meeting where she committed her life to Christ.

"I first professed when I was a child. My brothers and sisters all went to church. I was young. Mother told me just to be sprinkled.

"I was so small, but I never was satisfied because they were immersed, and I was just sprinkled. After I got married, we came back home and I asked our preacher, I said, 'Brother Angle, why can't I go down to the river here and be baptized today? I always wanted to be immersed.' So he put on my daddy's pants and we went down to the river. My family and my neighbors came down there, and I was baptized right down here in the river."

At a hundred and two, Sophia continued to read and listen to the Bible being read.

"I read the Bible a lot and I say the books of the Bible. Do you know the books of the Bible?" she asked me.

"I know there're sixty-six. Thirty-nine in the Old Testament and twenty-seven in the New," I answered.

"Yes, well, that's good. Do you know the names of all of them?"

I hesitated. "Maybe."

"Well, let me name them for you. Genesis has fifty chapters, Exodus has forty . . . ."

She went on to recite all sixty-six books of the Bible and the number of chapters in each book—a marvelous fete in my estimation. When she got to the end of the Old Testament, I challenged her to see if she could pick up in the middle. "How many chapters did you say Psalms had?" I asked.

Without flinching she said, "One hundred fifty."

"Are you sure?" I asked. "A hundred five or a hundred and fifty?"

"A hundred fifty. Here's a Bible. Look it up."

I did. She was right. She did the same thing for the New Testament.

I tested her again. "What is the shortest verse in the Bible?"

"Jesus wept."

"That was when Lazarus died, wasn't it?" I asked.

"Well, I guess it was when he saw Mary weeping. Lazarus' sister."

I checked that out when I got home. Sophia Dodson Hale had just taught me a Bible lesson. Jesus had not wept when first told that Lazarus had died. He shed tears when He saw Mary crying over the loss of her brother. Jesus had joined in with the family grief. He comforted Mary by shedding his own tears.

Contented And Happy

That her life had been pleasing was apparent from looking and talking with Sophia Dodson Hale. Her marriage to Escol lasted over seventy years. She still spoke of him as though he were there by her side.

"The fifteenth of February he'll be a hundred and one. I'm a year older."

They had two children with only one surviving to adulthood. She lost a brother in World War I. He died from pneumonia on a ship crossing to France (See the chapter about J. P. Ross). All of her brothers and sisters are dead now except one, and her husband died in 1985. Yet she maintained a thankful and cheery attitude toward life.

Although obviously intelligent, and with a sharp mind and memory into her hundred and third year, Sophia did not relate her happiness to her education or wealth. As men measure those things, she had little of either.

"I went to the eighth grade. That's as far as I got. I started to high school in Sparta, but they had an outbreak of measles. I had to quit. Back then, you had to board in town or stay with a relative if you wanted to go to high school. It was too far away to go back and forth."

A neighbor boy, Oscar Russell, who was three months younger than Sophia, rented a room in Sparta with some friends and continued in school, but Sophia had to drop out. That neighbor boy who grew up and lived on adjoining farms lived past a hundred also. (See later chapter)

Sophia enjoyed good health all of her life.

"I never was in the hospital until I broke my hip in 1986. Then I had a bout with pneumonia a few years ago. I eat about anything I want to. I like vegetables, fruits, and milk."

What does she do with her time now?

"I like to watch a little television. 'Wheel of Fortune' and some of the television preachers.

"Mainly, since my husband died, I've been making quilts."

She has four grandchildren and ten great-grandchildren for whom she made three quilts each. She didn't stop there, though.

"I'd say I've made over a hundred quilts since my husband's been gone. I'm getting so blind now that I can't see to do much."

Although some of her faculties may have been beginning to fail her when I visited on that February morning with Sophia Dodson Hale, her spirit was unflagging. More than most of us, she knew where she had been and where she was going. Quilting took her back to that joyous occasion when she met her husband in 1913, and her faith let her behold her future.

She looked me square in the eyes and quoted one of her favorite passages from the Old Testament. Psalm One Hundred.

"Make a joyful noise unto the Lord, all ye lands.

"Serve the Lord with gladness: come before his presence with singing.

"Know ye that the Lord he is God: It is he that hath made us, and not we ourselves; we are his people, and the sheep of his pasture.

"Enter into his gates with thanksgiving, and into his courts with praise: be thankful unto him, and bless his name.

"For the Lord is good; his mercy is everlasting; and his truth endureth to all generations."

"Don't we thank Him for the truth and the mercy?" she said in both a question and declaration.

Sophia Dodson was the sixth-born of twelve children of her parents, Harvey Mansfield Dodson b. 1-13-1860, d. 6-30-1946, and Betty Ann McCormick b. 7-26-1862, d. 6-27-1957. Grandparents were Jesse Dodson b. 1814, d. 9-21-1873, Mary Caroline Earls Dodson b. 4-12-1826, d. 10-10-1903; and Nelson McCormick b. 2-17-1830, d. unknown, and Elvira Clandenstine Myers McCormick b. 7-8-1836, d. 2-12-1896. She has one child, Geneva Hale Hayes, and one child who died at about one year of age. She has four granddaughters, ten great-grandchildren, and one great-great-grandchild.

Sophia Dodson Hale died November 11, 1993.

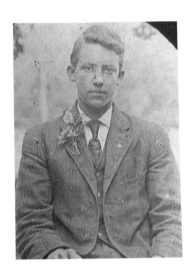 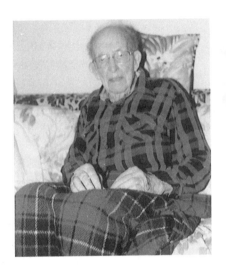

George Ray Gadd
Bledsoe County—March 10, 1893

L arge families were not rare in the late 1800s or early 1900s, but Ray Gadd had a distinction that few others could claim. His grandfather had twelve children, his father had twelve children, and Ray followed in the tradition by fathering twelve of his own.

Children in rural turn-of-the-century America were the same as wealth. They provided more hands to till the fields, milk the cows, chop the wood, tend the garden, and keep the house.

Large families provided the offspring with the opportunity to develop socialization skills that an "only" child from another family might not have. Did this necessity of having to get along in such large families have anything to do with living to an old age? More about that in a later chapter.

Ray Gadd lived in one of the more remote places in rural southeast Tennessee. When I drove from Interstate 40 to U.S. Highway 27 south to Dayton (historic location of the Scopes Trial) and turned off at Graysville to go up Grayton Mountain, I tried to imagine how that road may have looked eighty or ninety years ago. The tight switchbacks and curves that cut up the edge of the mountain were no easy task to navigate in a modern car on paved and maintained roads.

On the far side of the mountain would lie the beautiful Sequatchie Valley. But here, perched on the wind-raked flatland at the top, was his home at the end of a lane named for him. Ray Gadd still lived within a mile of where he was born. I was beginning to see that many of these old people had developed a sense of place from which they didn't wander.

I came to see him within a month of his hundredth birthday. He lived in a daughter's home and was tended by another. The sons and daughters were justly proud of a father who had worked at many different occupations to support such a large family.

What was Ray Gadd? I could have asked and received many answers. A sawmill operator. A farmer. A school bus driver. A father. A husband. A member of the Seventh Day Adventist Church.

But those were only parts of the answer. He would have said, "Just an ordinary man doing what he had to do."

Yet, while I traveled East Tennessee to talk with these ordinary men and women who in their own eyes were nothing special, I saw something extraordinary. They were the building blocks upon which communities, towns, states, and nations are built.

Their legacies may not be in what historians write about

them, and their memories may pass from this world with their grandchildren or great-grandchildren. But these were Tennesseans and Americans who were the glue that held things together so that others could be Presidents, and governors, and whatever. These men and women produced the wood, grew the food, and drove the school buses for our students.

And no one represented that better than Ray Gadd.

Ray Gadd and the people around him displayed toleration and acceptance early in the Twentieth Century perhaps better than is done now. Two examples illustrate that.

When women's suffrage came, the Gadd household joined in. His wife, May, was a Democrat while Ray was a Republican. Sometimes they canceled each other's vote out, but they voted.

In the small community, there were Baptists and Seventh Day Adventists. By an acceptable accommodation they shared one building. The Baptists worshiped on Sunday while the Seventh Day Adventists kept the original Sabbath on Saturday. I have not heard of this type of shared arrangement recently.

In talking with those who came to maturity in the early part of this century, I heard more stories of religious toleration again and again. In some places, the revivals by the Methodists and Baptists were scheduled so that everyone in the community could attend both, which they did. That would be rare today.

Ray Gadd remembered when he was a youngster the school session was for a period of three months. His first school seat was an old milk churn turned upside down. He wrote on a slate tablet with chalk. Years later he would haul children to a modern school as he drove their school bus.

Electricity didn't reach this remote mountain until 1946. Ray remembered electricity, the telephone, and refrigeration as being the most significant inventions and changes over his lifetime.

A trip to Graysville of eight miles was an all day affair

back when he was young. The mountain contained the coal that fueled the coke plants of the town, but the winding and steep road was dangerous.

It was little wonder that he stayed near home with his wife of sixty years until her death in 1973. Their twelve children were Lawrence, Martha, Margaret, Freida, Ethel, Edna, Betty, John, Donald, Clifford, Clara, and Bertha.

Society in this area has now changed from one based primarily on agriculture to one of service industries and small manufacturing concerns. The coke plants are history. And in this day and age, an abundance of children is neither necessary nor convenient. None of Ray Gadd's children carried on the tradition of having a dozen offspring.

Ray Gadd married Olive May Cunningham on March 16, 1912. His parents were Ancle Monroe Gadd and Mary Marshall Gadd.

Ray Gadd died October 16, 1993.

A Sense of Place

ill Jarnagin, Sophia Hale, and Ray Gadd (and most of the others that follow) lived their entire lives within a tight circle of a few miles. Mr. Jarnagin and Mr. Gadd lived within a mile of their birthplaces. Sophia Hale lived not far from her birthplace and practically at the place that she called home for a hundred years.

"My wound is geography. It is also my anchorage, my port of call," Pat Conroy wrote in the opening lines of *The Prince of Tides*.

We are tied to the land. We are citizens of the world. But more than that, we are residents of the United States, the South, Tennessee, and finally down to the community we call home. A sense of place is a sense of home.

Home is where the heart is. A house is not a home. Home is the place where, when you have to go there, they have to take you in. Be it ever so humble, there's no place like home. *Look Homeward Angel*. Many poets and writers over the ages have described the pleasures of home to us with these words and others. It is a place of rest, anchorage, and salvation.

Over the centuries, humankind has revered the ancient places of their ancestors or of great events. There must be an innate sense of place in us that tells us there's an importance in knowing where you're from—and why.

"Remove not the ancient landmark, which thy fathers have set," the writer of Proverbs tells us. Pilgrimages are made to the Holy Land for religious reasons for the Christian. Jews, Christians, and Muslims all consider Jerusalem a Holy City.

On the sectarian side, many people journey to historical sites in the country—to Philadelphia where the Declaration of Independence was signed, to the museums in Washington to view the ancient documents of our country, to the battlefields of the Revolutionary and Civil Wars. Others seek the places of their "roots" in England, Scotland, Italy, France, Germany, and the countries of Africa.

Is there within us an inbred sense of wanting to return to the places of our creation—physical, political, and religious—just as the salmon and the Monarch butterfly migrate over huge distances to their places of birth?

Certainly, in the centenarians who are part of this book, there was a strong tendency to stay near the place of their birth or return to it.

Estele Janeway had traveled to Alaska on construction and tried his hand at gold mining. But when I caught up with him near his ninety-ninth birthday, he was living within a mile of where he was born.

Oscar Byrd Russell, who was born a neighbor to Sophia Hale, had also traveled widely. In World War I, he went to Europe. He had lived in Texas, New Mexico, and Ohio, but when the Depression hit, he came home to White County, Tennessee. When I talked to him, just a month after his hundred and second birthday, he was living within a few miles of where he was born.

Psychologists and other professionals who deal with stress in people, tell us that moving from one home to another is one of the most stressful things in a person's life. It ranks right up there with divorce, death of a loved one, loss of a job, and health problems.

If a person's living habits naturally reduce stress, does that tend toward a long life? In these cases, these long-lived individuals stayed near the anchor of their homes. There must have been something reassuring about waking up each morning and being familiar with their surroundings, knowing where the nearest store was and who their neighbors were.

You will notice as you read the mini-biographies, these centenarians came from an agrarian society. Over and over again, they tell stories of working on the farm. Of course, ninety and a hundred years ago, Tennessee's population was mainly rural.

The Depression did not affect most of these centenarians all that much because of their agricultural roots. When Oscar Byrd Russell got laid off from his job at the tire plant in Ohio, he returned to the farm.

"Oh, we got by." "We had food." "No, things were tight, but we raised things," these centenarians said repeatedly about their experiences with the Depression.

While farming was hard work in the time that they grew up, fingernail-biting stress was not present. They pretty well knew where the next meal was coming from, and they could get by with fewer clothes or shoes. Because they made a lot of what they wore and grew most of what they ate, the farm was almost self-sufficient.

These centenarians were not, for the most part, globe-trotting high society. They knew their place and enjoyed it. It was on the farm, and it was home.

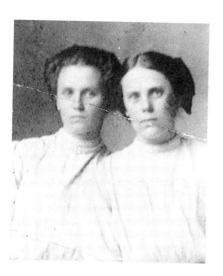
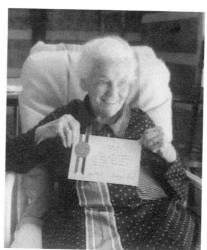

Mattie Cole (on left with sister Virgie) and near her 100th birthday

Mattie Smith Cole
White County—June 27, 1889

Mattie Smith Cole had been a resident of Sparta Health Care Center for over thirteen years when I stopped in to see her. I was there to see another person I had heard about when the nursing attendants told me about Miss Mattie.

"You'll just have to see her," they said, "but don't tell her we said she was over a hundred years old."

In fact, Mattie would be the oldest one that I had talked

to at that time. She was nearing a hundred and four.

She and another lady were talking.

"Mattie Cole?" I asked, looking at one and then the other.

She acknowledged me and invited me to take a chair. The other lady wandered from the room.

"I'm doing some stories on folks who are over a hundred. Are you that old?"

"I'm eighty-nine," she said.

I looked at my notes and information the other ladies had given me. I turned back to her. "You were born in '89. You're over a hundred."

"Who told you I was over a hundred?" she asked and brushed back silvery hair over her ear.

In what used to be called a nursing home, a place that many often think of as a warehouse for the feeble and dying, Mattie Cole still possessed an air of dignity and beauty. She had already proved to me that she was master, or mistress, of her domain.

Daughter of a furrier who would spend weeks away from home trapping and hunting, Mattie Smith grew up in White County as self-reliant as a young lady could be. She was born the fifth child of ten. She had five brothers and four sisters. She remembered their first house as being made of logs and having three or four rooms.

The arrival of the Model T was a time of excitement in the family. Transportation meant a little more freedom and movement around the backroads that were either dirt or mud, depending on the weather.

She never worked outside the home or held a "public job" as people of that age worded it. She married at the age of twenty-two and reared three children.

After Tennessee was the thirty-sixth and last needed state to ratify the amendment giving women the right to vote, Mattie accepted the opportunity but never ran for office or did anything in the way of politics other than voting.

The short visit convinced me that here was another Tennessee treasure. Mattie Cole had handled and could handle anything that came along.

Mattie Smith Cole was born June 27, 1889, fifth of ten children of John Buchanan Smith (b. 2-15-1854, d. 10-16-1918) and Mary Jane (Mollie) Jones (b. 10-21-1858, d. 12-30-1936). Grandparents were John Smith and Patsy Millsap Smith; and Eddington Jones (b. 11-10-1820, d. 8-30-1862) and Frances Jane Wisdom Jones (b. 7-9-1826, d. 3-5-1886). Mattie married Roe Cole on December 31, 1911. They had three children: Irene, Waymon, and Thelma. At the time of my interview, Mattie Cole had living nine grandchildren, sixteen great-grandchildren, and fourteen great-great-grandchildren.

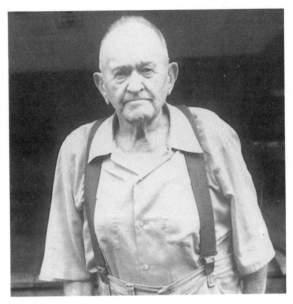

Henderson Estele Janeway
Grainger County—November 21, 1896

S ometimes it must be good luck, providence, or something like that which allows these centenarians to live to their extraordinary ages. Estele Janeway is a prime example. He could have died at half his age if he had been a little more miserly.

In the mid-1940s he traveled to Alaska to work. His visits there eventually took him to the gold fields where he formed a partnership and tried his luck with the rich mineral. But he remembers the time he almost didn't make it back to Alaska after a trip to Tennessee.

"I went to Alaska on the boat, but every trip after that I came out on a plane.

"On one trip I went over to the airport to buy my ticket

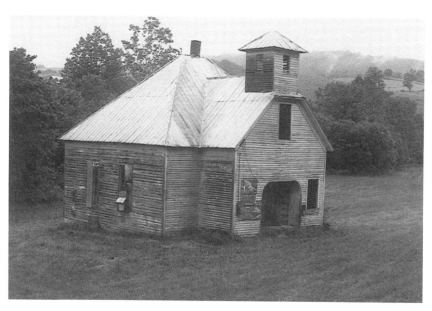

An old school house near Estele Janeway's home

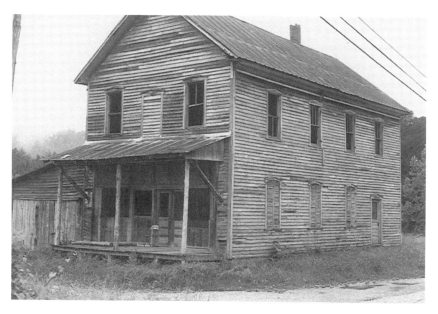

Deserted early 1900s general store building

and asked how much it would be to Seattle. They told me I could get a plane ticket for thirty-five dollars cheaper and get there five hours later. It'd go a different route.

"I stood there a minute and said, 'Give me the first one that'll get there.' The one that would have saved me thirty-five dollars fell out there in a pasture field and killed everybody on it.

"That's the one I'd been on if I'd tried to save thirty-five dollars."

I had been given Estele's name by a relative two years before I ever got around to going and seeing him. So many of the ones that I was going to see had died between the time I received their names and found time to go see them. When I called his home, though, he was still around and invited me out.

Estele, born in Grainger, lived within a mile or so of his childhood home—in Union County right on the corner of where Claiborne, Union, and Grainger meet. Apparently none of the three counties took responsibility for the roads near his house.

It was a rugged part of the county that had changed little in the past hundred years. The setting was one that a film maker would have chosen if he had wanted to depict the Tennessee hill country of the early 1900s.

I turned off a paved road onto a narrow gravel lane that took the most direct route up a ridge and over. The wheels on the rear of my little pick-up spun as they tried to find traction in the wet gravel. The road narrowed even more when I crossed the crest of the ridge and started down between two ridges that paralleled the road.

With rain pouring down, I watched for the house that had been described to me. There ahead on the right a faded-white clapboard perched beside a swiftly running stream that had been swollen by the rain. A swinging bridge crossed the stream, leading to Estele's front door. I stepped out and back in time eighty or so years.

A crusty old man, Estele sat attired in blue jeans, suspenders, and a shirt opened wide at the neck. He was a different centenarian from many I had talked with. He had been through the wide stretches of the country and worked at construction on many projects. But like most of the others, he had a sense of place, and settled into a house not far from the place he was born to spend his final years.

He didn't mince words. I asked him what invention of the Twentieth Century had changed his life the most. He said he didn't know, but he knew what had cost him the most.

"I'll tell you what cost me the most—getting rid of the first damn woman I had."

Estele had been married three times, although he only counted two—the one he had such a difficult time "getting rid of" and the one who died. The third hardly mattered. He would have forgotten her except for the reminding by his companion, Edith.

"My second wife died around 1932," he said.

"So, you haven't been married since then?" I asked.

"No."

"Yeah, you did. You married when you came back from out yonder. It didn't last," Edith said.

"I don't figure that. It just lasted two weeks," Estele replied.

"I thought when you said 'I do'—you do," Edith said and had the last word on the subject.

Estele was the youngest of six children. His father died before Estele's first birthday, leaving Estele's mother to fend for four boys and two girls. They survived by farming the hilly farm land. His mother, Martha Myers Janeway, never remarried and died in 1951 at the age of eighty-four. She was a young widow of thirty when she was thrust into being the head of a household which had children from a year old up to twelve.

As far as Estele can remember, there were no grandparents on either side around to aid the family. "No, I don't even remember them. I don't even know their names now. I forgot." Is it unusual then that Estele grew to be a rather independent and foot-loose individual?

He attended the typical one-room school of that time. One similar to the one he went to still stands—deserted and weatherbeaten— within a couple of miles from where he lives. An older brother and sister both taught at one time or another at the school during a span when teachers were not required to be college graduates but only had to pass an examination.

He learned to drive a bulldozer and operate heavy equipment. Following the construction and oil industry, he worked at various times in Kansas, Oklahoma, Oregon, and Alaska. "I've been from here to near the North Pole." He spoke from beside his bed in a room that was cluttered with furniture and the items of daily living.

Estele's military career was cut short by the fact that he had gone to sign up on the day that World War I ended. "I liked about twenty-four hours getting into the Army. I got to Rutledge to sign up. They gave me my dinner and learned that the Armistice had been signed. They sent me home. A bunch of us boys were there ready to go."

When he came back to East Tennessee from his far west wanderings, Estele opened a "beer joint" in Knoxville not far from where the old Market House stood. It was called the V Grill.

"Did you drink very much?" I asked.

"I've never smoked, and I never did drink much."

"You sold beer, but you never did drink very much?"

"No, I didn't taste it for five and a half years. Them fellows would come in and ask to buy me a beer. I'd tell them no. They'd buy it, but not me. I didn't drink it."

At his heaviest, Estele said he reached one hundred ninety pounds. "I use to be five foot nine inches. Now, I don't know. Your old bones wear down."

What is his daily routine now that he is in his hundredth year?

"I get up late. I watch television until about midnight.

Watch the late news. I'll go out and get the wood we need or just piddle around. I don't do too much."

What does a hundred year old eat?

"I'm not too particular. I don't like tomatoes for one thing. I don't eat much meat. I like vegetables and fruit. I like sweet stuff. I like butter."

"He'll eat butter on butter," Edith interjected.

Although the past century has brought much change to the state and country, Estele's surroundings harken back to a past era. Electricity only came to his little valley in 1953 although the Tennessee Valley Authority's Norris Dam is less than twenty miles away. It was completed in the early 1930s.

Yet, he remembers the early days as being even rougher.

"The roads then went up one hill and down the other. In the winter time they were so muddy you couldn't hardly get through.

"Our house had four rooms downstairs and two up. We had two big fireplaces that we heated from. Used wood like everyone back then did."

Estele Janeway still drives when he wants to. He started driving before he had to have a driver's license but has kept his all these years. He has four children spread out from California to Knoxville.

He is not married to Edith, in whose house he lives. They explained that her deceased husband and Estele were best friends. Estele came to visit when he heard that Edith's husband was sick.

"I came here to help her with the work when her husband got sick. He died. Then I got sick, and she brung me here. When I got well, she got sick, and I helped to take care of her."

Looking at Estele Janeway, I knew I was seeing a man who had enjoyed his hundred years. His explanation of his living arrangements was not necessary.

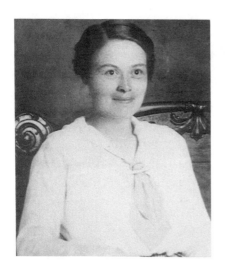 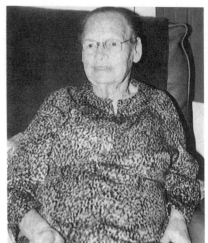

Jennie Dunaway Raby
Knox County—June 7, 1894

Jennie June Dunaway Raby's life is a study in contrasts. She was born in Knox County just across and up the Clinch River a mile or so from where Oak Ridge would be built in the 1940s. Yet she remembers the area when there was no bridge across the river, and they had to navigate the water in little boats she called "skittles."

"The roads were so bad you couldn't hardly get in here with a wagon, let alone a car."

But she wasn't afraid to hop aboard cars when they came along. Her parents had warned her about riding with anyone in one of those new-fangled machines. However, when she and a sister were walking back from another relative's and they were offered a ride by a couple of men in a Model T, they took it.

"I didn't think nothing about it. I just got in, and after I did, I was scared to death. But then they just let us get out where we told them we wanted to. But I got to studying what they had always told us at home."

Before cars, the train was what Jennie and her family depended on for transportation back and forth to Knoxville. It came by at nine in the morning and left Knoxville at five in the afternoon.

Born the middle child of nine, she remembers the family moving across the river to the Freels Bend area of Anderson County early in her life and the little village of Scarborough Town. Now, all of that is part of the Oak Ridge reservation that took up much of the valley. Then, though, her father farmed the Freels' rich bottom land and did handyman work to eke out a living.

"Over there is a chair my father made. He was real good at wood work. My husband was too, but not as good as my father."

Then when the whole family went back across the river, they could take a ferry boat that was pulled along a cable by manpower. Beaver Creek, where she was born, wove its way from above Powell Station through northwest Knox County and powered different mills, including Couch Mill. There the Dunaways had their corn ground.

When all the scientists and construction workers came to work on the Manhatten Project at Oak Ridge, Jennie was more concerned with raising her family. She had married in 1917 at the age of twenty-three to a man she met at Chandlersview Methodist Church. He was a widower with two children. Then they had six of their own children beginning in

1919. Four of those lived to adulthood.

If those weren't enough, Jennie's sister and her husband died, leaving five children. Jennie and her husband took them in.

It's probably little wonder that her favorite invention was the washing machine. But before that there was the scrub board. "We washed on a washboard. There was a big family of us and it took a whole lot of rubbing on one."

What was happening on the other side of the river, in what was later to be known as the Atomic City, affected the Raby family very little from a practical standpoint. They would never be able to farm the land of Freels Bend again, and perhaps the work in Oak Ridge which led to the ending of World War II was as welcomed by the Rabys as by anyone else. But more than anything, it marked a passing of an age.

Jennie Dunaway Raby was born into the horse and buggy age, and then she was transported into the atomic age although she had never lived more than six miles from where she was born.

She saw her role as homemaker—a job that took all her energies and attention. When women's suffrage came along in 1920, Jennie Raby was little moved.

"Did you get out, register, and vote?" I asked.

"No. I never did vote in my life. My husband always voted. I always thought that was the men's place."

She says it without embarrassment or apology. She didn't mind that other women did vote. Her patriotism and contribution to the country revolved around her family. Others would have to deal with the problems outside that realm—there were enough within her family circle.

Her firstborn child, Zelma Louise, died in 1920 at the age of seven months. One sister died in 1921 at the age of twenty. Jennie's mother, Margaret Parlee Dyer Dunaway, died on May 11, 1921. Her father, Lewis Wesley Dunaway died August 19, 1922. Another sister died in 1923 at the age of twenty-five. A third sister died in 1929. The 1920s were marked with grief everyplace she looked. Voting just did not seem that important to her in the larger scheme of things.

Three and a half months after her firstborn died, Jennie gave birth to another child who is the oldest of her living children. She had three more who survived to adulthood and then a final child in 1934 who died at birth.

As inevitable as death and dying is, Jennie has done an admirable job in handling it and adjusting to it. Sometimes, like the 1920s, it seems it was thrown at her in bunches. In 1973, her husband died in April, and then she lost a brother and sister within a month later in the year. She is the last survivor of her brothers and sisters, and three of her children are dead.

While her family was the center of her life, Jennie felt for those less fortunate than herself. The step-children and nephews she helped to rear speaks to that. But she almost tears up when talking about those who were displaced when the Oak Ridge project began.

"I knew a lot of them. One poor old man used to live across the river there. He didn't live no time after he left his home."

The farm life meant raising animals and killing them for food and hides, but Jennie couldn't bear to kill even a chicken.

"We mostly just bought what we couldn't raise. We salted the meat down and hung it. It would last all summer."

"Did you kill your own chickens?" I asked.

"Not me. I wouldn't kill them. Somebody else in the family would have to do that. I stepped backward one time on a hen with a bunch of little chickens and killed a little bitty baby chicken, and that liked to have killed me."

Jennie claims that she has "been nervous" all her life. That was her main ailment. She suffered a broken shoulder in the mid-1970s which didn't heal properly, preventing her from raising her arm above her head. She has problems with acidic foods, but otherwise she eats what she wants.

When I talked with Jennie June Dunaway Raby, she

was still going to church on a regular basis and looked forward to everyday.

"I get up about seven or seven-thirty."

She divides her time helping about the house where she lives with a daughter, Flossie Raby, making quilts, and helping her daughter make saddle girths.

Her large family includes thirteen grandchildren, twenty-eight great-grandchildren, and eighteen great-great-grandchildren.

She never voted, she never drove, and she never flew. She is one of the last of a breed of the frontier woman who met adversity and death head on and never flinched.

Jennie Dunaway Raby's parents were Lewis Wesley Dunaway, b. 7-17-1856, d. 8-19-1922, and Margaret Parlee Dyer Dunaway, b. 12-23-1867, d. 5-11-1921. Grandparents were Leroy Dunaway, b. 1826, d. unknown, and Mary Cagley Dunaway, b. 1833, d. unknown; and Isaac Dyer, b. 1840, d. unknown, and Debby Maples Dyer, b. 1840, d. unknown.

A Sense Of Family

L o children are an heritage of the Lord: and the fruit of the womb is his reward.

"As arrows are in the hand of a mighty man; so are children of the youth.

"Happy is the man that hath his quiver full of them: they shall not be ashamed, but they shall speak with the enemies in the gate." Psalm 127.

"Children's children are the crown of old men; and the glory of children are their fathers." Proverbs 17: 6.

Practically all of the centenarians in this book came from large families. Cora Arnwine had six brothers and five sisters. The same was true for Ray Gadd. Mattie Cole had five brothers and four sisters, the same as Sophia Hale. William Gault is the record holder with fourteen siblings, twelve of whom lived to adulthood. Ruth McCollum, Mary Conley, and Jack S. Humphreys had fewer siblings than the average.

Most came from families averaging over eight children. Along with brothers and sisters, there often were other relatives (aunts, uncles, or grandparents) who lived with them or nearby. (See chapter on Socialization Skills)

The family is the oldest and smallest unit of society. Before there were communities, towns, cities, states, and countries, there were family units.

How does family help to account for the ability to live to an old age?

For one thing, it shows that these men and women had mothers and fathers (mothers especially) who were healthy and vigorous. Childbirth was difficult, dangerous, and usually attended only by midwives at the time most of these centenarians were born. Good genes go a long way toward a long life.

Families provided their own miniature communities where these children grew up. Again, mostly in a rural, agrarian society, these families functioned often as self-contained, self-sufficient cells of society. Children quickly learned their places and their responsibilities.

Being near grandparents, uncles, and aunts who could relate the oral history of the family to these children also could have aided in imparting to them a sense of purpose and belonging. A sense of usefulness in the family unit that continued through adulthood often provided the impetus for looking to the future with a higher expectation that things would work out.

While these centenarians came from parents "whose quivers were full" of children, they did not follow their example. The women whose stories are told here came from families with an average of eight children. However, when they became mothers, they averaged having only four children.

What is the story here? While having a large number of brothers and sisters may have been useful in developing skills that led to a long survival, the same was not true for having a great number of children.

Childbirth was still physically draining and depleting when these centenarian ladies were of childbearing age. Repeated childbirth can wear a body down to where it is more susceptible to disease and earlier death.

Do these families' histories prove that out? Although I wasn't able to obtain the age at death of some of these centenarians' parents, the average mother's age at death of the ones I did obtain was 79, and they averaged having eight children each.

All of these men and women, except Grady Haynes and Tom Garland Wallace, had children—just not as many as their parents. The exceptions are Ray Gadd and Mary Conley. He was the father of twelve. However, his wife, the mother of these twelve, died at 78. Mary had ten children.

The family unit was preserved by each of these centenarians as they reached adulthood. All married. Except for two, they all stayed married to the same spouse until the spouse's death. And, of these, none remarried following the spouse's death.

Family consisted of a father and mother, grandparents, brothers and sisters, a spouse for life, and children.

The tradition of strong family relationships continued through their children up through the times that I talked with them. The majority were either living with a son or daughter, next door to them, or within a short distance.

The unit of the family, instituted in the beginning, was a sustaining force in making possible the long lives of these men and women. From their births, they encountered strong and caring groups of relatives. This they perpetuated and nourished through their own families of spouses and children.

Although the families became smaller, the sense of care, concern, belonging, and looking forward remained.

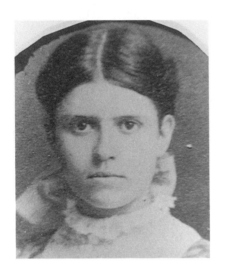
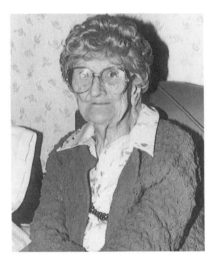

Rosa Mae Stamps Sliger
Putnam County—February 7, 1892

T he sounds of music washed against the walls of the house with the regularity of the rising evening tides of oceans far away that she never would see. The coming of the hundred-dollar organ to her house was a highlight of Rosa Mae Stamps early life in Putnam County, Tennessee.

"I could make that thing sing. We'd all gather around it and sing. Hymns and Christian songs. Sometimes I would sneak in something I heard someplace else. My mother would look around the corner and say, 'Where did you hear that?' "

When I talked with Rosa Mae, less than a week past her hundred and first birthday, her eyes sparkled when she talked about music and the "happy family" she had as a child and adult.

Both sets of Rosa Mae's grandparents lived in the

Calfkiller Community of Putnam County southwest of Monterey. Now, Interstate 40 passes the outskirts of Monterey, but at the turn of the century, the grandparents still used oxcarts for transportation.

They would go to either Verble Baptist Church or Johnson Baptist Church. The children would ride or walk barefooted until they got near the church building, then stop, wipe their feet off with cloths, and put on their shoes before entering the house of worship.

Rosa Mae's grandmother, Mary Jane Finley, was barely eighteen when the Civil War started. As the war progressed, bands of Confederate soldiers would pass through Putnam County, often scavenging for food and supplies.

Mary Jane owned a beautiful horse and was afraid of losing him to the roving units of soldiers. She took him to a nearby cave and hid him there anytime she thought the soldiers might be passing through. It worked for a while, but one day she entered the cave looking for her sleek horse to find he had been replaced with a worn out nag.

Rosa Mae was born the fourth child of seven to Anderson Stamps and Frances Henry Stamps. She was the first girl born to her parents after they had three boys. She had two younger brothers and a younger sister.

"Tell me about the organ," I said while we sat in her room at the Cookeville Health Care Center. "Where did you get it?"

"Bought it. They had them here in Cookeville then. There's a store that had all kinds of them. Dad came in one day and said, 'I got a surprise for you.' I said, 'What in the world is it?'

"When they came driving up there with that organ, oh boy was I happy!"

"How old were you?"

"I was fourteen."

"Did you learn to play it right off?"

"No. It took me three days to learn to do a thing on it.

Nobody showed me a thing about it. I believe, if anything, the Lord helped me. We'd play it about every night until ten o'clock."

One thing she regretted when she married Clyde Sliger in 1912 was that they could not afford an organ.

But even when she went back after marrying, she would play the songs her family loved. "All the whole family sang. People don't know how to do that now. It's a different life altogether."

For a couple of years, her father moved the family out to Oklahoma looking for work during the first decade of the century. There it was different.

"Oh Lord, you could see for miles and miles in Oklahoma. Level just as far as you could see. And there is—I call them ant hills compared to our mountains—little hills."

Rosa Mae also lobbied her father for other modern appliances. "One day I seen a woman washing with a washing machine. I said, 'Daddy, how much money you got? I'm tired of rubbing them clothes. Let's try a washing machine.' "

She also saw a refrigerator in town one day and told her father how good that would be. They had electric lights in Oklahoma, but when they moved back to the Tennessee hill country, they had to wait quite a few more years for electrification.

Rosa Mae and her husband settled into a married life which included voting together.

"My husband let on like he wasn't going to vote unless I went with him and voted too. He wanted me to go with him anyway. We were six miles from town, and we went horse back or by buggy."

She was happy that World War I didn't take her husband from her.

"No, he didn't have to go. He was scared to death, like all the others were, that he was going to have to go. But he had a medical problem, and they released him. Oh, that was one pitiful time. We all cried and prayed all night. So foolish that they can't talk things over and fix things up without having a war."

Rosa and Clyde had eight children—five boys and three girls. She went from one big family to another.

"Wherever there was one, there we all were right there together working or no matter what we were doing. If we were singing, we all were singing. If it was eating, we all were eating together. At night we had our prayer and Bible reading."

Before I left, I commented on her doll collection and her colorful flower print dress. She said she had a boyfriend who visited her, and she had to pretty up for him.

"May I take your picture?" I asked.

"Sure. But my boyfriend might get jealous."

Life was simple for Rosa Mae—simple, sweet, and rich.

Rosa Mae Stamps Sliger's parents were Anderson Stamps, b. 6-15-1860, d. 5-22-1936, and Frances Henry Stamps, b. 3-11-1867, d. 9-21-1938. Her grandparents were Jasper Henry, b. 5-23-1832, d. 9-10-1924, and Mary Jane Finley Henry, b. 11-24-1844, d. 12-13-1920; and John Stamps and Julia West Stamps. Her children were Vestal, Hazel, Jerry, Odell, Cecil, Lester, Louise, and Mary.

Rosa Mae Sliger's daughter passed on to me some old phrases which she said were from her grandparents' time and are becoming unknown and obsolete to this generation. Some of them are:

Banking the fire; chunk up the fire; skim the cream off the milk; work the butter; scour the water buckets; fill the fire box; poke the fire; render the lard; tie a broom; stripping fodder; making bats for a quilt; carding the cotton or wool; slopping the hogs; setting a hen; getting the milk from the spring; churn the milk; put on a back stick; making molasses; and drying pumpkins and green beans.

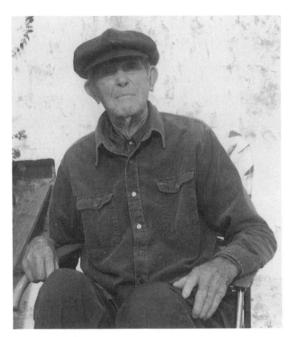

William Albert Gault
Knox County—July 14, 1893

T he reluctant warrior turned into the grand marshall of Knoxville's Veterans' Day parade in 1993. It wasn't that William Albert Gault didn't want to serve his country, but instead, the twenty-four-year-old would just as soon have stayed home in his native Tennessee when he was drafted.

However, if they wanted to have a parade and let him ride in the lead car, he would be glad to wave and smile at the now diminishing crowds who had any interest in remembering wars or the soldiers who fought them.

He pointed to the picture of him at the parade and smiled. "Yeah, I wouldn't have been in the war if they hadn't drafted me. When they discharged us, they tried to get all the men to re-enlist, but I wouldn't do it for any price. I wouldn't do it."

Those who sought to glamorize or glorify war hadn't talked to the likes of Sergeant Alvin York or William Albert Gault. They did what they thought they had to do. There was nothing about shells exploding and bullets whizzing overhead that enticed either to stay any longer than they needed to.

"The twelfth of August (1918) we loaded on ship in New York and went straight north. It took us twelve days to go across. They done that to dodge the submarines. They wouldn't mess with us in that ice. So, we had five thousand men on the ship, a French vessel, and you had to have all your winter clothes on or you'd freeze out on the deck. We went in between Ireland and Scotland and then to Liverpool, England.

"We stayed in England two or three weeks and then went to France."

"Did you get into any of the fighting?"

"No. I was in the 81st Wildcat Division of the light artillery. We did a little practicing. It took four horses to pull that gun and a little cart behind it."

Just four months before Albert Gault had crossed the Atlantic by the northern route, a Missouri Army artillery man by the name of Harry S. Truman sailed a similar course and also ended up in France for practice before going into battle.

Author David McCullough in his biography of the President, *Truman*, describes what Albert Gault must also have witnessed on that crossing: "The weather was clear the whole way across, perfect submarine weather. The ship was part of a convoy, sailing a zigzag course once it reached the submarine zone. . . . The water was either blue or lead-colored, he noted, depending on whether the sun was out or in. The only variety in the panorama came at sunrise or sunset, and the sunsets weren't half as good as back home."

When November eleventh came and the Armistice was announced, there was joy and shouting all along the front and back in France where Albert Gault and his artillerymen had been preparing for war.

Albert Gault wasn't the first in his family to go to war. An uncle, his father's older brother Tom Gault, fought in the Civil War.

"His foot's over at Norris at the museum," Albert Gault told me, referring to the Museum of Appalachia at Norris, Tennessee, directed by that inveterate collector, John Rice Irwin.

"He was in the Civil War and lost one foot. I don't know which one it was, right or left. I think he fought for the South.

"I don't think they bothered his leg, just his foot. He had a thing he buckled around the calf of his leg and had a shoe made and sized. I don't know which leg it was. He lost his foot and they had to take it off above the ankle."

In talking further with Mr. Gault, I tied down that it wasn't actually his uncle's foot that they had at the Museum of Appalachia, but the wooden prosthesis that was made for him after losing the foot. It is still displayed at the museum on occasion.

The other tale he remembered from his family about the Civil War was about visits to their house by soldiers passing through the east Knox County area.

"They had a log house. It wasn't awful big. It had a loft and attic. They kept bee hives in the attic above the loft. During the Civil War an officer wandered up and wanted a drink of water. They had those long-handled gourds. They got him some water from the well out in the yard. One of those bees stung him, and he thought someone was shooting at him. He spurred his horse and took off."

"Why did they keep bees in the attic?" I asked.

"I don't know. They also had a place under the floor in the first room where they kept the honey down in there."

The Gaults farmed on the east side of Knoxville near the French Broad River before it meets the Holston to become the Tennessee in the area known as Straw Plains or Strawberry Plains. He remembers as a youngster crossing part of the river to farm a little island. "Five or six acres there, I guess. We had near a hundred all together. Raised corn and hogs, a little of most everything else."

It was there in east Knox County that young William Albert Gault went to school under Dora Kennedy, an extraordinary educator who later had a school named for her. His education ended with the eighth grade although he had a brother who went on to high school.

Albert was the fifth of fifteen children born to James Henry Gault and Cora Larue Gault. Twelve of the children lived to be adults. The children were spread out so that some were grown and gone from the home before the last ones were born.

"We had a big fireplace that had an iron rod to hang pots on that would swing in over the fire to cook with. I guess the fireplace was six feet wide."

The family's moves included those to other farms around the forks of the rivers and then to Anderson County where they farmed near the Claxton Community.

"There wasn't more than a third of it you could tend. Bull Run Ridge you couldn't do nothing with."

Before the United States entered World War I, Albert tried his luck farther west.

"I stayed out in Kansas City all winter and worked at a freight depot. In the spring I went up to Iowa, and there's where I registered for the Army."

After the war, he rejoined his parents in Anderson County before acquiring a place of his own in the Lonsdale area of Knoxville.

His first Model T gave him a broken arm. "Well, the engine died, and I didn't flip the switch. You had to crank it by hand. When it caught, the crank flipped back on me and broke my arm. I went to Doc Cobb. He fixed me up, and I never had no more trouble out of it."

Lonsdale became too much like a city to him, and he found an opportunity to get back out into the country.

"I traded it to S. B. Newman Printing Company for a place down here (near Snyder Road in West Knox County)."

It was after that move that he married Viola Mae Ruckart in 1928. Leon was born the next year and a daughter, Frances, in 1935.

As the state and nation paused for the Great Depression, he sold out in Knox County and moved back to Anderson County. There, just a couple of years later, TVA began the Norris Dam project, and Albert went to work helping to clear the land for the dam and reservoir. He worked for TVA by night and tended his corn fields by day.

Mr. Gault ate about anything he wanted except for pork and a few things that upset his "over-acid" stomach.

"Don't you like pork?"

"Shoot, like it? I like it better than a drunk likes liquor."

The doctor had told his mother to take him off pork when he was a young child because of stomach problems. He eats fish and some beef. Peaches are his favorite fruit, and he has a strong craving for sweet potatoes.

He drove until he was ninety-four, but now he allows his son or daughter to take him places.

I stood to go and asked him to let me photograph him. He motioned to go outside to one of his favorite places beside his house on Ball Camp Pike.

He buttoned his large corduroy shirt, eased his cap down over thick hair, and sat facing the warming sun of a late November afternoon.

Maybe I was the only one who noticed the symbolism. The reluctant warrior turned his face away from the East and war, and in the late November of his own life, sat back comfortably in his chair and took in the rays of the sun. He was the ideal warrior who did his duty and then turned back to help build his country, looking westward.

Albert Gault died March 30, 1995, at his home.

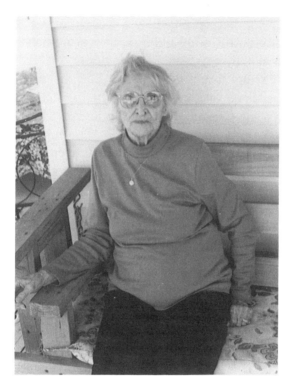

Cora Beeler Arnwine
Grainger County—December 29, 1895

A wedding by the river wasn't originally planned, but that's the way it turned out. The oldest of twelve children born to Alfred and Carrie Beeler, Cora was only fifteen when she decided to marry into the Arnwine family of Grainger County. Both families had been in the area a long time, some in Grainger and some across the river in Claiborne.

"I was always afraid of water and fire. Those are two things I stay away from," she said some eighty-odd years after the marriage. But that fear didn't keep her from crossing the Clinch River to marry Clarence Arnwine when she was fifteen.

"My mother didn't know I was going to get married. We were going to slip off and marry. But my husband and his cousin passed by my grandma's house on their way to Claiborne County to get the license. She caught on to it.

"She came and told my mother that Clarence and his cousin had gone over there to get the license. She begged me not to get married."

Since her husband obtained the license in Claiborne County, the couple had to be married in the same county.

"He got a preacher from Liberty Hill. He and his wife came across the river in a little boat. We did too. We just went across to the other side so we would be in Claiborne County. Family came and watched. Some could see it from the Grainger County side of the river.

"We went back to my husband's folks' house to eat dinner. The preacher and his wife came up there too."

Before that marriage, Cora helped on her parents' farm which was typical of East Tennessee at the turn of the century.

"I hoed a little corn. We raised a little bit of everything. Chickens, hogs, sheep, goats, and horses. They had a sawmill on the farm and sold logs and lumber."

And when her father accumulated an abundance of large logs, he would take a trip.

"They'd put the logs somehow down near the river. When the river got up—Clinch River—they'd take the logs, tie them together, and build a little house in the middle of the logs so they could cook and eat. Then they'd float all the way to Chattanooga.

"Weren't no dams then. They'd get to Chattanooga and sell the logs and come back home."

I looked at the map and checked the route her father and the ones like him must have taken on the Clinch to Chattanooga. They would go by where Norris Dam is now, on past Clinton, past the area where Jennie Dunaway Raby lived as a child near what is now Oak Ridge, then down to Kingston and past my back door to meet the Tennessee. It must have been an arduous task to maneuver the logs along the river for over a hundred and fifty miles without power of any kind except for long poles. They depended on the current of the river for propulsion.

I had heard other old East Tennesseans tell similar stories. The Clinch and Tennessee Rivers were arteries of commerce. The rafts of logs had to go with the flow of the river. When the Clinch met the Tennessee at Kingston, they continued on toward Chattanooga instead of turning upstream on the Tennessee to go to Knoxville. Lumber was a cash crop long before tobacco became so important.

Cora attended school and church near where she grew up. "There was a Methodist Church and a Baptist Church both near us. The Methodists would have their church in the morning, and the Baptists would wait until afternoon. They'd both get the crowds that way."

The problem with school was the lack of books.

"We used the same books over and over. I went four years in the same books. I quit. I guess I just got tired because of them four years in the same books. Over and over again."

Cora's family, through her grandmother, did pass along some oral family history of the Civil War.

"I heard them talk about the Civil War. They buried some of the valuables in the graveyard so the soldiers wouldn't take them. The soldiers would bring their horses through and just turn them loose to eat our corn and grain. They'd come in and cut the feather beds up, looking for valuables.

"On my father's side, he had a brother that fought in the Civil War. A band of soldiers caught him and hung him for some reason. I don't know why. It was David Beeler's brother.

"My grandfather on my mother's side—Charlie Brooks and his two brothers were in the war. I'd hear tell of some of them being captured and they put them behind a fence to keep them.

"They didn't have nothing to eat. When the old horses died, they'd have to eat horse meat. It was awful to hear them talk about it."

Cora's husband, Clarence Arnwine, did a bit of farming and horse trading to make a living for him and the three children that were born.

Cora didn't know everything about her husband.

"How much older was your husband than you?"

"To tell you the truth, I never did know how old. You know, the war came up, and his brother changed his name so he wouldn't have to go to war. I changed it back. I don't know how old he was."

Cora's husband developed kidney trouble and died in 1925, leaving her a twenty-nine-year-old widow with three children. She had been married half her life, but she went back home. She worked on their farm in the tobacco that was now making its presence felt in East Tennessee to a larger extent.

"Some people raised tobacco, and I worked in that. I could really tie that 'baccer up. But it was hard work.

"My mother told me to go to Middlesboro. They had an overall plant there. I worked there for several years. I went to Knoxville and took a beauty course and opened a shop."

When Cora spoke of Middlesboro, I asked if she knew any of my kin there. It turns out she had been treated by Dr. Cawood.

"I went to every doctor in Middlesboro. I went out of town to a country doctor. I tried everything. I had bad gas to where I had to sit up to sleep. I couldn't lay down.

"Dr. Cawood told me, 'Let me tell you one thing. You can stop eating too much grease. Cut your grease out and your gas will be gone.' That's all he said. It worked.

"I told my mom that everytime she cooked something to let it get done before she put the seasoning in. I'd get mine out before she put the seasoning in."

It was pleasing to know that my cousin had relieved her gas pains.

Later Cora had to have two operations for gall stones and a bad appendix. "I went to the doctor. They took x-rays. Those x-rays don't show up nothing. I guess they think I was fooling them. They finally found out my gall bladder was bad and took it out."

Cora Arnwine survived as a single parent during the 1920s, the Great Depression, the 1940s, and until now by being a gutsy woman who wasn't afraid of work. From clothing mills, she became an entrepreneur. Her three daughters gave her seven grandchildren and many more great-grandchildren.

She moved to Roane County to live between Harriman and Rockwood with one of her daughters. She is within eyesight of Interstate 40 that knifes up Walden's Ridge to the west.

"I like to eat anything that comes along. I don't care much for sweetened stuff."

Cora enjoys traveling to another daughter's in El Paso. "I've been traveling around pretty much, out there around New Mexico, Texas, and Louisiana. No, I don't fly. I go by car."

She enjoys the changes that time has brought but doesn't regret the hard times of the past.

"Oh, it's changed awful. Back in them days you didn't have no kind of music except a banjo or fiddle. It's been years since I've been back to where I was born. When I moved, I got used to people. I got used to the new places."

Cora Beeler Arnwine's grandparents were David and Tilda Beeler; and Charlie and Catherine Brooks.

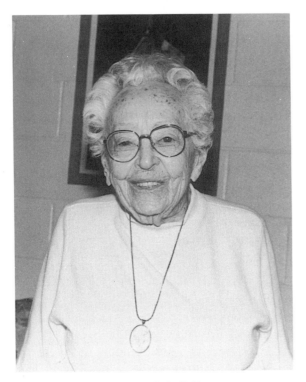

Pauline Hill Massey
Etna, Tennessee—September 3, 1896

A violin, the influenza epidemic of 1918-19, and evangelist Billy Sunday. These three entities—so different in nature—came together in an odd coincidence to introduce Pauline Hill and her future husband, Bill Massey. But let's not get ahead of the story.

Born the second child of William Walter Hill and Lula May Hill Hill, Pauline's earliest memories are of mining camps where her father practiced medicine up and down the Sequatchie and Tennessee valleys.

The now non-existent town of Cardiff in Roane County is where she spent her younger years. "My father practiced medicine from Rockwood up to Emory Gap all along the valley."

Pauline had an older sister and a younger brother and sister. The children's births spanned a period of eighteen years.

"My father was born in White County and my mother in Roane County, as best I remember."

Most of her life was lived in Harriman, although she lived several years in Cardiff and Chattanooga.

"I started school down there in Cardiff, but they found out that I wasn't learning much. So, my parents sent my older sister, Ivy, and me to Harriman to live with my grandparents—my mother's parents—Isaac and Margaret Kindrick Hill during the school year so we could go to school in Harriman."

Harriman, the City that Temperance Built, was just a child itself when Pauline and Ivy came to live with their grandparents and attend school. Established in 1891 as another idealistic experiment, the town did have good schools and new houses.

Her father and mother soon moved to Harriman to live in a nearby house on the corner of Carter and Cumberland. Her father gave up the general practice of medicine and became an eye, ear, and throat specialist. "What he did mostly was test eyes and make glasses. He did very little surgery."

Pauline began to attend Mooney's Academy which had previously been a boys' school. Then she went on to Harriman High School, graduating twice—first when it only went through the eleventh grade and the following year when they added the twelfth.

"Now, I never did go to college. I got interested in the violin, and I went to Chattanooga and studied under Professor Cadek. He was a very, very noted violinist and was a wonderful teacher."

Most of the time, Pauline traveled back and forth to Chattanooga on a weekly basis for her violin lessons. Very few things interrupted that routine—only the flu epidemic of 1918-19.

"The flu epidemic was awful. People just died like flies. There was a scarcity of caskets in Harriman to use for the dead. My father gave up his regular practice of medicine and went from street to street, house to house, treating the sick."

(Over 550,000 died nationwide during the epidemic. Statistics are not available for the small towns and counties of Tennessee, but at least 550 died in Memphis and another 350 in Nashville. These were directly related to the flu, but many others died from complications of the respiratory affliction. A good guess would be at least 10,000 over the state. In the military, troop ships were hit with the outbreak. Hundreds died on the ship that J. P. Ross was on.)

Across the street from Pauline Hill lived the Crain family.

"Mr. Crain came to our door one day. He said his wife could not eat anything. She had the flu really bad. What were we eating? My mother told him that I had fixed some rice and would be glad to take some to his wife if he liked.

"Mrs. Crain was one of the sickest people that I ever saw. Her doctor had told her not to drink any water. She was burning up. I crushed up some ice and put it to her lips to cool her mouth.

"They had a big pot-belly stove in their house, and it was hot enough to kill you in there. I said, 'You need some fresh air.' She said, 'The doctor told me not to raise the window.'

"Well, before I left, I raised it a little to cool the room off. The next day she fired her doctor and had my father treat her. He let her drink all the water she wanted.

"She later referred to me as her 'Little Angel Of Mercy' for the help I had been."

After Mrs. Crain recovered, her family and her in-laws went to Chattanooga to attend the services of Evangelist Billy

Sunday. Pauline Hill was also spending the summer in Chattanooga studying the violin. It was on that trip that Mrs. Crain introduced Bill Massey (her sister-in-law's brother) to her "Little Angel Of Mercy." Bill Massey and Pauline Hill were married in 1922. So, it was through the coincidence of the flu epidemic, her violin lessons, and Billy Sunday's presence in Chattanooga that Pauline met her husband.

They lived in Chattanooga from 1922 through 1927 while Mr. Massey worked for the Southern Railway. It was in Chattanooga that their daughter, Kay, was born in 1926.

The family returned to Harriman where the city had just the year before voted to have Tennessee Power provide the town with electricity. Bill Massey went on to be an owner of the Harriman *Record* newspaper and later to be postmaster for twenty-five years.

Pauline occupied her early married years with giving violin lessons to Roane County children and rearing her daughter and her son, Charles. She later became the attendance teacher for Harriman High School and worked with the parents and students to keep them in school.

She began driving in 1920, the same year that women received the right to vote. "I did both. I drove when you saw very few women driving. I drove more than my husband. I registered to vote as soon as I could. Now, that's one thing I've always done. I think it's our duty. Now that I live here in Johnson City, it's harder to learn about the local candidates. I voted in the last Presidential election. I helped put Bill Clinton in. I may help put him out this time." She laughed.

"I saw my first car when I was ten. The first radio I listened to, we had to use earphones.

"I've seen a lot in my lifetime. I've been to the Holy Land twice. I stood near the Cape Canaveral launch site and watched some of the first astronauts go up."

Except for childbirth, Pauline has only been hospitalized one time. She has no special diet and eats about anything she wants.

Exercise has always been a big part of her life. "I used to walk five miles along the beach when I visited my daughter in Florida. I played tennis until I got too old. Then, I took up golf. I played golf on my 95th birthday. We started an exercise group for older people in Harriman called Body Recall. It was great for us. I quit driving when I was 95 because of my vision."

Pauline and her sister, Nancy Pearl Hill, gave up housekeeping at their ancestral home in 1993. They moved to the Appalachian Christian Village where they have separate apartments. She remains active there and talks with friends who drop by. Besides her two children, she has five grandchildren and fourteen great-grandchildren.

"I take plenty of vitamins but no flu shots."

Pauline Hill Massey's parents were William Walter Hill, b. 10-24-1861, d. 12-1-1955; and Lula May Hill Hill, b. 12-6-1871, d. 1-4-1959.

Putting Grief In Its Place

All of these centenarians lived through times that could have been emotionally damaging to anyone. The Spanish-American War, World War I, the Great Depression, World War II, the Korean War, and the Vietnam War have all occurred on the national and world scene during their lifetimes. The influenza epidemic of 1918-19 took many of their friends, neighbors, and family.

On a personal level, these survivors have seen parents, brothers, sisters, spouses, and children die. They have suffered economic and health setbacks during their lives that would have staggered others. Have they found a secret to dealing with grief and putting it in its place?

Most of these centenarians are religious. They believe in a Higher Power. They see purpose in events or, at the least, believe that someone greater is in charge.

Perhaps they do the same as King David did when his first son by Bathsheba died. His servants were astounded that David wept and fasted while the child was ill but bathed and ate after the child's death.

"Then said his servants unto him, 'What thing is this that thou hast done? Thou didst fast and weep for the child, while it was alive; but when the child was dead, thou didst rise and eat bread.'

"And he said, 'While the child was yet alive, I fasted and wept: for I said, Who can tell whether God will be gracious to me, that the child may live?

"'But now he is dead, wherefore should I fast? Can I bring him back again? I shall go to him, but he shall not return to me.' " II Samuel 12: 21-23.

David's next son by Bathsheba, Solomon, wrote these words in Ecclesiastes:

"To every thing there is a season, and a time to every purpose under the heaven:

"A time to be born, and a time to die; a time to plant, and a time to pluck up that which is planted;

"A time to kill, and a time to heal; a time to break down, and a time to build up;

"A time to weep, and a time to laugh; a time to mourn and a time to dance." Chapt. 3, verses 1-4.

These centenarians, more than most, have learned these lessons. They are not unfeeling individuals but ones who have learned the "times" and "season" for the emotional lows and highs of life. *Season* means that there is a set amount of time, a limit, for these emotions to be expressed. Then there is also a *time* when they are appropriate.

More and more the medical profession is learning and admitting the ties between emotional well-being and physical well-being. *Psychosomatic* was a term not used so much a hundred years ago. Yet, the phenomenon was there.

Jennie Dunaway Raby probably provides the best example of living through grief. During the 1920s, she lost her first-born child one year, a sister and mother the next year, her father the following year, another sister the next year, and a third sister a few years later in the same decade. Then in 1973, her husband died, and then a brother and sister passed away later in the year.

She coped with all of the deaths and grief in her own way. She was not callous or uncaring, but she didn't dwell on who died. She focused instead on who was living. She had children, nieces, and nephews to rear.

She had feelings for them all and for those she didn't know all that well. In talking about a farmer who was displaced when the government bought his land to build the Oak Ridge plants, tears filled her eyes. "I knew a lot of them. One poor old man used to live across the river there. He didn't live no time after he left his home."

Jennie Raby, while a prime example of dealing with grief, certainly is not alone among these men and women. None of them went unscathed through a hundred years of living.

Dealing with grief was handled nobly by all these centenarians.

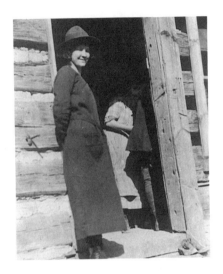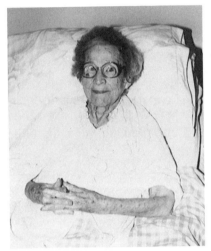

Kotolene Holt visiting a neighbor and later at home in Farragut

Kotolene Hamilton Holt
Sullivan County—April 18, 1896

S trawberries, horses, and shoes for the winter. Those were the memories that flooded the mind of Kotolene Holt when I asked her to tell me how things were in her childhood in upper East Tennessee.

Born the seventh of nine children to William Ellis Hamilton and Lura Tennessee Milhorn Hamilton, Kotolene's main job on the farm in Sullivan County in late spring was to pick the strawberries. They were one of the cash crops that her father used to support the large family.

The nearest town was Bristol. The farm lay along the bank of the Holston River. Most of it is now covered by Boone Lake.

"I was raised in four rooms with the front of the house being logs. In later years the old log house was torn away and a new front built to the house. It had six rooms then where all of us lived."

Shoes for youngsters in those days were worn from frost in late fall until the sun of spring warmed the grass and ground enough that the children could go barefoot.

"Oh yes, we couldn't wait to take off our ragged shoes in the spring. We went barefooted until frost."

With nine children, her father didn't find it feasible to take them all to Bristol, sixteen miles away, to buy shoes in the fall.

"My mother would take a twig from a tree and measure each of the children's feet. She put a twig, broken to the size of each child's foot, in a bag for my dad. He would take that bag to Bristol and come back with another bag full of shoes.

"We had a time going through that bag to find the shoes that fit all nine of us."

For recreation as a child, Kotolene cared equally for dolls and horses. "I had an upstairs where I'd sneak up there by myself and play with my dolls for hours. When I was through, I put them back in the wardrobe where no one else knew where they were."

But for rough and tumble play with the boys, there was nothing better than going into the pasture and riding the horses bareback and without a bridle.

"My brother who was about eight years older than me loved to ride the horses. I learned from him. I got to be about as good as him. We'd just go out, catch a horse by its foretop, run, and jump on.

"We had a favorite horse, and it got to be that when he saw us coming, he'd run to us so that we could ride."

Her childhood was a time before washing machines and refrigerators.

"We washed clothes on the washboard. We'd use the rainwater we caught, or if we were running low on that because of washing vegetables or whatever, we'd go to the pond and do the washing. It was a big pond between our two barns."

Cooling of milk or butter was done at the spring house.

"It was down over this steep bank down in the valley. We'd put our milk and things we needed to keep cool in there. It was a good spring."

Her family were Methodists. Over a hundred years before her birth, Bishop Asbury had ridden horseback into the southern area of Virginia and planted the seeds of Methodism in the frontier. The Sullivan County area was still strong in that tradition.

Kotolene took to school. School was about a mile and a half from the house. It was an easy walk. She finished grade school, high school, and then went on to what is now East Tennessee State University.

At twenty-one, she passed the teachers' examination and took on her first school. At first she just had the lower three grades. Then later, she had a school with eight grades and about twenty-five pupils.

She showed me a picture of one of her schools. Some of the children appeared older than eighth graders. She looked again at the photo.

"I know they look older. They were. They didn't go through school as fast then as they do now."

She started teaching before World War I. Only her younger brother Sam served in the armed forces.

"Sam was younger than me, and he joined the Navy. He made three trips to France to bring the soldiers home from the War."

After she married on January 30, 1923, she left teaching and helped her husband on a farm not far from where she grew up. They had one child, Ruth, with whom she was living in

Farragut when I talked with her.

When they started building the dams and making the lakes that would give the valley electricity, Kotolene's life, like many others, changed.

"It was theft. They took part of my farm. What the lake took up came up might near the house. That was the prettiest view along the lake where our old house was."

Electricity came to her home in 1946. It, along with the automobile, she saw as the greatest instruments of change in her lifetime.

The farthest Kotolene traveled from her East Tennessee roots was to Atlanta to live with her daughter after breaking an arm when she was eighty.

She saw television as a mixed blessing.

"How happy we were to get that first television. But how the Devil used the airways after that! But we were sure glad to get that first one."

In her last years, Kotolene left television because of impaired hearing. She still read. With the large print editions, she found happiness in reading stories of far away places or words of inspiration from the *Upper Room*.

She held near her eyes the photo of her and the twenty-four school children she taught when she was in her early twenties, a smile graced her lips, and for that moment I could tell that she was back with them doing what she loved.

Socialization Skills

A nother phenomenon that goes hand in hand with the large families that these centenarians came from is the interaction they had at an early age with a large number of people from disparate age groups.

The average number of children in these families was eight. Ages of the children varied widely. Some of the first ones were grown and gone from home before the last ones were born.

Aunts, uncles, grandparents, and cousins abounded, either in the home or nearby. They had to learn to get along, to share, to wait, to do without, to help, to laugh, and to cry at an early age.

A few years ago there was a book titled *All I Really Needed to Know I Learned in Kindergarten.* These centenarians didn't have kindergarten, but they had family—an abundance of people—all around. It was no place for a recluse or for someone who shirked his or her chores.

Psychologists and those who deal with family counseling tell us that personalities are often related to the birth order of the child. A first-born often has different characteristics than a middle or last-born child. Traits of aggressiveness or accommodation may be tied to the child's order of birth.

The centenarians whose stories are related here had six first-borns among them. Ray Gadd and Cora Arnwine were both the first of twelve children in their families. John S. Humphreys, Grady Haynes, and Mary Conley were first-born but had fewer siblings. More of the centenarians fell into the middle-born category.

A middle-born child not only has the parents and grandparents and uncles and aunts who are older but must learn to deal with siblings who are both older and younger. When there are only three children, the middle one might feel lost in the lack of his parents' attentions. However, when there are a half dozen or more children, the situation may be different. While the oldest and youngest probably hold special places in the family, numbers two through five may, as a group, become more accommodating and less competitive.

The oldest daughter almost becomes another mother at an early age in families with numerous children. These daughters were often given responsibilities beyond their chronological ages. On the other hand, the oldest son was the first one to go to the field, barn, mill, or store with his father. He, like the oldest daughter, would acquire characteristics of maturity beyond his years. While these abilities may afford success in the business world, the built up stress of having these responsibilities thrust upon a child may, in the long run, lead to the same debilitations as other stressors. However, the six first-borns in this book displayed a remarkable ability to overcome any stress and live to a ripe old age.

W. A. Gault said that although he was the fifth of fifteen children (twelve living to adulthood), some of the older brothers and sisters were grown and moved out before the youngest ones were born. They weren't all in the home at the same time except on special occasions.

Estele Janeway was the last-born in his family because his father died within a year of his birth. He and J. P. Ross are the only last-borns among this group. If any child in birth order is the special, pampered, and privileged child, it is usually the last-born. But in the case of Estele, this would not have been so since he would have had to assume responsibilities of a man early on after the death of his father.

As far as birth order goes, middle-born children did better in living to old age in this small sampling of centenarians in total numbers, but the number of first-borns (six) is quite significant. The middle-born has the ability to relate not only to his or her adult parents but also to siblings who were both older and younger. Perhaps they acquired earlier than others abilities to mediate and make peace. The first-borns, on the other hand, were able to overcome any stress related to their early maturity and function as adults sooner and with great durability.

Socialization skills acquired at a young age undoubtedly helped these centenarians cope with the world throughout their long lives.

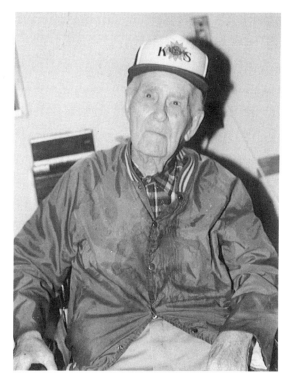

Oscar Byrd Russell
White County—January 15, 1891

T here must be something in the spring water in the area of White County where Oscar Russell and his neighbor, Sophia Dodson Hale (See pages 7-15), grew up and lived near each other or on adjoining farms off and on for a hundred years.

Oscar was just three months younger than his neighbor. He was a month past his 102nd birthday when I talked with him in Sparta in February of 1993.

Jobs, World War I, and the depression took Oscar on a circuitous journey from White County to Texas, New Mexico, Ohio, and then back to Tennessee. Of all the centenarians who appear in this book, he is among the most traveled. However, as was so common with the others, when I saw him, he was living within ten miles of where he was born, grew up, and lived the majority of his life.

He was the second child of William Matthew Russell and Emma Lewis Russell. He had four brothers and three sisters.

In his youth, the extended family included a grandmother and others who lived under the same roof from time to time.

"We lived in a two-story log house. It had about seven rooms in it. Dad always raised sheep. He liked mutton. My grandmother took the wool and used it."

School was just for a four-month term. To attend high school, he had to rent a house in Sparta so that he would be near the only high school.

In 1910, at age nineteen, he went to Texas to seek his fortune, or at least to try to make a living with his older brother, Walter. He worked as a streetcar conductor and also in the fire department.

When World War I came along, Oscar signed up with the Navy and spent two years on a supply ship going back and forth to France.

When the War ended he returned to Dallas to join Walter. They bought a restaurant and tried that for a while before he moved to New Mexico with his wife, Bessie Haston Russell. There they homesteaded property the government was offering to veterans about seventy-five miles from Albuquerque.

"I had a little farm. Mainly grew beans. Had about six head of cattle. It was okay as long as we got rain. But when it didn't rain, it was hard to make a living. Sometimes there wasn't much rain, but in winter there were the biggest snows. Three feet deep one time."

It was in New Mexico that he bought his first car. And

it was the proliferation of automobiles that led him to his next employment. He moved with his wife and young family to Akron, Ohio, where he worked in tire manufacturing until the Depression hit hard.

While the Depression made money scarce, Oscar, like many farmers, knew that he could at least survive on the farm in White County. In 1930, he and his family returned to the constant of his early youth where self-sufficiency on the farm was a way of life. He didn't leave again.

Instead, he built up a quality herd of Hereford cattle on a farm that grew to 179 acres that included land adjacent to the farm of Sophia Dodson Hale.

Oscar and his wife had two children (Emma Russell Boyd and Paul Russell), four grandchildren (Janet Boyd Hill, Karen Boyd Henry, Paula Russell Polk, and Dr. Mark Russell), and several great-grandchildren.

On his Hundredth Birthday in 1991, one of the guests was Sophia Hale who gave him a special quilt, one of the many she had made over the years.

Oscar Russell died October 19, 1993, just twenty days before Sophia Dodson Hale.

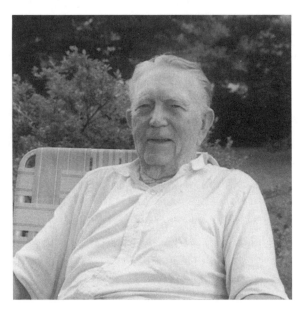

Jesse Philip Ross Sr.
Greene County—December 9, 1896

T he girl at Walmart looked at my driver's license and said, 'This can't be right. It says you were born in '96, and we ain't even gotten there yet.'

"'That's 1896, my Dear,' I told her. Then she says, 'You're 96-years-old? And still driving?'

"I said, 'Yep. I aim to keep on driving until I get too old.' "

J. P. Ross laughed when he told me that story. He sat in an aluminum lawn chair in his large yard beneath the shade of an ancient oak tree on a sunny summer's day. On his place just a couple of miles from downtown Harriman, he had weathered the years of his life in fine spirits. He could look beyond me and see the house his father had bought in 1919, and a little farther to the garden he tended daily.

"I want you to go back up to Greeneville with me. I'll show you where I grew up. It was different back then."

J. P. was the last of six children born to George Washington Ross and Melindi Florence Willett Ross.

Like many in the Southern Appalachians, Ross believed his heritage to be rooted in the Scots-Irish tradition, along with English. His father and paternal grandparents were most likely born in North Carolina—in or near Yancey County.

"Grandfather Ross was captured by the Confederates in the Civil War and accused of being a spy. They could never prove anything. He was probably guilty because he was a strict Union man all right. He wouldn't have been past slipping around a little information if he had it.

"He lost his health in prison and died. I never did see him."

The institution of indentured servitude played a role on his mother's side of the family.

"The story I got on my Willett side is that they came from England and my great-great-however many greats back-grandfather was bound to service to a family named Willett. They more or less adopted him, and he took on the Willett name."

Ross remembered that they used coal oil lamps when he was growing up.

"We didn't always have the dime to buy the gallon of oil, or we didn't want to walk the two and a half miles to get it. Then we'd use a grease light."

"What's a grease light? How did it work?" I asked him.

"You just took a vessel and put some grease in it. Hog grease was good. Then you'd put a piece of cloth in it for a wick and light it. You could use a cake pan or a pie tin—just any kind of metal vessel to hold the grease. It worked."

President Andrew Johnson had been a tailor in

Greeneville before his ascendancy to the Presidency. He died in 1875, twenty-one years before J. P. Ross was born in the same town.

Ross worked on the first paving crew that turned the streets of Greeneville to a more solid base for automobile traffic.

"I set the first curb and gully forms for the first paving in Greeneville. Church Street. It started right at the railroad tracks. That was before World War I."

Before the time of automobiles, J. P. remembered taking a blind horse hitched to a wagon to his brother's wedding.

"I was just a kid. I was going to my oldest brother's wedding. For some reason I ended up with the old blind horse at our house. They had taken the good buggy horse. There weren't any rock roads. When it rained, they were just mud and mud holes. There were little holes that the wagon wheels would drop into and rock the wagon. There were bigger holes that you'd want to avoid.

"Anyway, I was on this road with a blind horse pulling the wagon down a muddy road with holes in it. I came up to a hole, and I didn't know whether to let the horse step into it or try to get him to go around.

"I finally opted to keep him going straight. He hit that hole, his feet slid out from under him, he went down, and the front part of the wagon rolled over him. It was a mess. I jumped out, unhooked the traces, and got him out from beneath the wagon. We both were as muddy as we could be."

They had ten grades of school in Greeneville, and J. P. had finished nine of them before his first job and the war.

He was just the right age for war but was fortunate in that he never saw any battles.

"I was in the engineering corps—148th Engineers. Our primary job would have been to build pontoon bridges. We'd go in front of the army when it was advancing and follow it when they were retreating. We put the bridges down and took them up.

"I went to France on the USS George Washington. There were about 10,000 of us on there. More than a hundred died of the flu going over."

Within a month of his reaching France, the Armistice was signed ending the war. However, the engineering corps stayed on for another ten months or so. He helped prepare the stadium where Olympic-type games were played.

He was in Paris when he came close to one of the big generals of the war—John J. Pershing.

"I was in Paris and they had a review of our company near the stadium. After they dismissed us, I just wandered around like a young boy and came near the General's car—it was called a LocoMobile—with his chauffeur sitting in there. I just looked around. Then General Pershing comes up. I snap to attention and salute. The General salutes back, gets in his car, and they drive off.

"When I got discharged back to Atlanta, I went into a movie theatre, and there I was on the newsreel standing next to the General's car and saluting!"

Although he didn't fire a shot in the war, J. P. Ross later met the Tennessee hero of World War I, Alvin York, near his home in Jamestown.

"I was in the wholesale grocery business. I used to run into him out there in Fentress County. I remember the last time I ever saw him. He was in a little country store there in Grimsley looking for black powder for his hog rifle. Used to you could go into most any grocery store, especially a country store, and buy powder and shot. Then it got so you couldn't get it, and he was out looking for powder for his rifle."

While J. P. was in the Army in France, his parents sold their place in Greeneville and moved to Harriman, about forty miles west of Knoxville.

Trying to find his folks' new home was how J. P. met his future wife.

"I had never been to where my folks moved. When I came back out of the service, I went to Greeneville for a while before going to Harriman. It was a time of travel by train. I had seen my folks in Greeneville and told them I'd be down on a later train.

"My brother was supposed to meet me and my cousin at the depot, but we were delayed. When we arrived around midnight, there was no one at the depot. It was dark, and I just had general directions to turn left over the railroad tracks and go up and around the hill.

"My cousin and I got a cab and pointed the driver in what we thought was the right direction. He drove around, stopped and asked people if they had heard of my folks. No one had since my folks were new to the area.

"We wandered around and finally went back to the Cumberland Hotel. I had a room upstairs and they put her downstairs. She was just about sixteen and was scared to death.

"Anyway, the next morning we took back out. I was walking down this lane where my parents lived and there was a house right off the road. A young lady was standing there.

"I asked her, 'Lady, can you tell me where I live?'

"She said, 'You must be Mr. Ross' son.' She pointed down the road.

"About two years later I married that lady that showed me the way home."

He married Edith Marie Davidson in 1923.

J. P. went back to upper East Tennessee for employment in construction and with the Greeneville engineering department before returning to Harriman during the peak of the peach growing craze in 1927.

"Within three years, the bottom fell out of the peach market. There was the Depression and no good transportation. If we had transportation like we have now, I could have made it as a peach farmer.

"There weren't any roads. You had to ship them and load them in an ice car and take them off up north on the train. You didn't know where they were going or how much you would get for them. Commission men would handle the sales. A lot of times I didn't get enough to cover the labor.

"The whole county was doing peaches. Kingston and all around."

Looking back over his near one hundred years, J. P. Ross said the greatest changes were in transportation and communication.

"Probably the most important invention was the computer. If you look at all the explorations we've done in space and whatever, without the computer, it would have taken a lifetime to have done the calculations.

"But for me personally, transportation and communication were the two things that changed most in my life time."

He and his wife had five children, ten grand-children, and at least that many great-grandchildren. His wife died in 1977.

When I talked with J. P. in late June of 1993, he maintained a robust life style.

"I hardly ever go to bed before 11:30 or midnight, and I usually get up around seven. I get out in the morning into the garden before it gets hot and work a little.

"I still drive, but I don't drive at night.

"I take the daily paper and local paper. I read the *Reader's Digest.*

"Oh, I like sports. Baseball and football. I'd like to have the Atlanta Braves as my favorite team, but it's disgusting how they play sometimes. I also watch the Chicago Cubs on television."

Jesse Philip Ross Sr. was the sixth child of George Washington Ross, b. 12-1-1853, d. 1942; and Melindi Florence Willett. His paternal grandparents were Jesse Helton Ross and Nancy Arwood Ross. His maternal grandparents were Phillip Willett and Caroline Johnson Spears Willett.

J. P. Ross Sr. died May 29, 1995, Memorial Day.

Minnie Ruth Griffitts McCollum
Loudon County—May 17, 1894

She was postmistress at Greenback for twenty-three years, but Ruth McCollum did not look upon that as any great accomplishment. She retired in 1950 at sixty-five.

"Sam, my husband, was to be the postmaster. But he said for me to take the test too, and if he didn't pass, I would. We both passed, but he insisted on me being postmaster. That way he'd have time to work there in the post office and on the farm too."

Longevity didn't run in Ruth's family, although her mother lived to ninety. Her father died at seventy-nine. Her maternal grandmother died at forty-three and maternal grandfather at fifty-two. On her father's side, her grandmother died at eighty-one and grandfather at fifty-nine. Three of her grandparents were dead before Ruth was born.

She remembers her then surviving grandmother Lucy Ann Burton Griffitts as being a religious woman.

"She lived near the National Camp Ground. She was a devout little lady. She gave us a prize of ten cents to memorize the Hundred and Third Psalm."

Ruth was the second of four girls born to John Burton Griffitts and Mary Louise McClain Griffitts.

"My parents were both Methodists. But when they settled there at Morganton, there was no other church close except a little Presbyterian church. We didn't have a good means of traveling. So they took us there and we were reared in the Presbyterian religion.

"My daddy was a farmer. He had a three hundred acre farm there on the Little Tennessee. He farmed all his life. He raised chickens and cattle. I helped with bringing in things from the garden. I would feed the chickens and gather the eggs. They didn't really require much of us girls."

Her childhood home was "an outstanding house at that time," she told me. "It was wood. Well built. It was a lovely house."

Much of her family's farm was taken into the Tellico reservation in later years with part of the farm being now beneath the lake.

Ruth married at nineteen and moved with her husband Sam McCollum to Blount County where they too had a farm of nearly three hundred acres. When the Depression came, they had less, "But we always had plenty to eat."

Ruth traced her ancestry to Scotland and Wales but knew little of their history. There was little oral family history passed down once her ancestors were assimilated into the New World and they became *Americans*.

She and her husband had three children. Howard was born in 1914; Esther in 1918; and Sam in 1921.

It wasn't until the 1960s when she was near seventy that Ruth flew in an airplane for the first time.

"My son-in-law had a little airport in Bryson City, North Carolina. He came over and offered to take me on a ride, and I went. He flew around over Maryville and Knoxville. He would ask me, 'Mother are you frightened?' And I would say, 'No,' but I was so scared. I knew I'd feel better when I got on the ground. But I enjoyed it."

"Back in 1920, when they gave women the right to vote, did you start voting?" I asked.

"Well, I just voted because they gave us that opportunity. I didn't do any fighting or anything to get that right, though."

From the time that her grandmother rewarded her with a dime for memorizing the Hundred and Third Psalm, Ruth McCollum became an avid Bible reader and student. "I'm on my sixtieth time of reading the Bible completely through. My faith in the Lord Jesus is the sweetest experience I've had, and I'm just looking forward to Heaven. Now, it's not the church, it's your faith in the Lord Jesus that saves you."

Minnie Ruth Griffitts McCollum's maternal grandparents were Joseph McClain, b. Oct. 10, 1838, d. March 15, 1882; and Ruth Euphemia Howard McClain, b. Oct. 7, 1838, d. Nov. 24, 1890; and her paternal grandparents were William Houston Griffitts, b. May 19, 1825, d. May 17, 1884; and Lucy Ann Burton Griffitts, b. Jan. 31, 1829, d. Feb. 16, 1910. Her parents were John Burton Griffitts, b. June 16, 1849, d. Dec. 4, 1928; and Mary Louise (Lucy) McClain Griffitts, b. Jan. 26, 1868, d. Aug. 12, 1958.

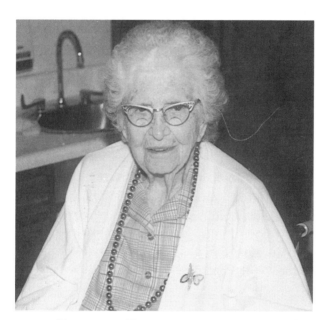

Leona Drews Turner
Indian Territory—Oklahoma—April 12, 1892

I worked and saved my money all my life to live in my old age, but I never expected to live this long," Leona Turner told me from behind twinkling eyes that illuminated an indomitable spirit. It was 1993. She was 101 and recently had her legs amputated because of poor circulation. Since both her parents died when they were fifty-three-years-old, she had no expectation of living close to their combined years.

"I went to Kansas City when I was in my early nineties by myself. I flew Delta. They were wonderful to me and helped me."

She was a late-comer to Tennessee. Born in Indian Territory fifteen years before it became a state, she moved with her parents to Kansas at about four years of age.

Leona remembered her Indian neighbors in Oklahoma. "The land was given to the Indians that were run out of this part of the country. We had neighbors who were Indians. They were very, very nice. There was not much for them to do. They couldn't raise anything on that ground. It was the poorest ground ever made."

Her father was a German immigrant. She remembers him as being very strict with his children (Leona's mother had thirteen and reared ten to adulthood). He insisted that they retain the use of the German language and discouraged them from going to the English speaking schools. Leona was forced to withdraw from school during her first year.

Not to be held back by her stubborn father, Leona taught herself how to read and write English. She believed her father thought that the German immigrants would come to dominate the United States if they retained their language and heritage.

Rather ironically, her father died in 1908 having failed to live long enough to see one of his sons fight in World War I against the German homeland or to know that two of Leona's sons would fight for the United States against Germany in World War II.

"My father died of black lung. He was a coal miner. My mother died of cancer. In those days there were not many doctors or hospitals. We hardly knew what a nurse was."

After she dropped out of school, Leona went to work and married when she was fourteen.

"What one invention changed your life more than anything else?" I asked.

Without hesitation she answered, "The washing machine," and then added, "and refrigeration."

In Oklahoma and Kansas where she lived ice was a precious commodity. "Now, we used to, if we wanted any ice, bring it home and put it in a big wash tub. We'd cover it with an old quilt or blanket so it wouldn't thaw as quickly."

Truman and Franklin Roosevelt were her favorite Presidents.

"I've seen his (Truman's) home. They showed it on television during the last election. He had a plain looking farm house. He came back home with the honor of not bothering anything or making any money on the government. The most he had spent of government money was to have the iron rail fence that ran around his house electrified to keep people out. I liked him very much."

Leona outlived two sons with only her daughter living when I talked with her.

Leona Drews Turner was not a native Tennessean like most of the others in this book, but she showed the same grit and determination and became another Tennessee treasure.

Leona Drews Turner died October 27, 1995.

Grady Haynes
Scott County, Virginia—October 31, 1895

G rady Haynes is another non-native of Tennessee who deserves mention among these centenarians. He lived a great deal of his life in Tennessee and was a graduate of the University of Tennessee Medical School at Memphis even though he was born in Virginia just across the state line from Bristol.

He was the first born of five children of John K. Haynes and Beuna Vista Harrell Haynes. They moved quite a bit when he was very young. From Virginia to Waco, Texas, and then back to Tennessee before he was five years old, they traveled.

Between the time he was five and six, Grady developed a form of osteo-tuberculosis which affected his left leg. The country doctor his parents took him to decided to consult with two specialists in a nearby town.

"The specialists looked at my leg, and they both recommended taking it off above the knee," he remembered over ninety-five years later. "The country doctor thought about it for a while, came and picked me up off the table, and carried me out. He told them he would try another course of treatment for a while."

At a hundred years of age, Grady Haynes still had his left leg. "I had to walk on crutches for two and a half years, but I was always thankful to that 'country doctor' for saving my leg."

With that experience in his memory, Grady Haynes went on to be a physician himself, specializing in the treatment of tuberculosis for several years after he became a doctor. Some thirty years later he looked up the country doctor who had saved his leg. He lived near Morristown, Tennessee.

"He was retired and sitting in a chair on his porch at a house on a country lane. I came up to him and said, 'You remember me?' He said, 'No.' I told him he had saved my leg when I was a boy of five, and now I was a doctor. Tears rolled down his cheek."

Grady Haynes was drafted into World War I but was released to return to medical school. He served in the medical corps in World War II with the rank of colonel.

Dr. Haynes worked at various locations during his long life. He married but had no children.

When I caught up with him in January 1996, at the Appalachian Christian Village in Johnson City, Tennessee, he was living in the same general neighborhood where he was born and reared.

Of Medium Build

I f these centenarians were asked, they all would probably
say they were just "ordinary people." They didn't see
themselves as special. In this sense, they were of medium
build.

It was also true in a physical sense. These men and
women tended to be of average build. There were no really
obese men or women, although a few were probably heavier
than the height and weight charts would have allowed.

None ever mentioned being on a "diet." Several said
that they didn't care much for sweets. A couple avoided tomatoes and other acidic foods. William Gault said he didn't eat
pork because of a childhood malady, but he liked it "like a
drunk likes liquor." Cora Arnwine said she asked her mother
to take her food out before she put the greasy seasoning in after
she had a bout with her gallbladder and stomach.

On the other hand, Estele Janeway said he really liked
butter, and he almost ate butter on butter. John Humphreys
didn't pass up the crispy-fried fat of a slice of ham. Most
mentioned a diet that consisted of more fruits and vegetables
and less meat than the average American eats now. This was
perhaps because of their economic circumstances in growing up
rather than a planned course of dietary control.

In short, their natural diet tended to be more healthy than most Americans enjoy today.

There was no mention of any exercise program. That is the good news. The bad news is and was that they worked hard. While there were no jogging trails, aerobic classes, stationary bicycles, or buns of steel video workouts, there were chores such as putting up the hay, washing the clothes on washboards, milking the cows, cooking meals for large families, carrying in coal and wood for the fireplace and stove, and numerous other tasks on the farm and in the house. Living, in and of itself, was a test of physical endurance.

Medicine and doctors were scarce for most of these centenarians, but there was an occasional need for a doctor, a hospital visit, or an operation. These men and women saw doctors as a last resort and took medicine for ills only when absolutely necessary.

Most of them were generally healthy all of their lives. John Humphreys had thirty-six years of perfect attendance at his Kiwanis Club and never missed a meeting of the Knoxville Board of Education during his twelve years' service.

The great influenza pandemic of 1918-1919 did not directly infect these men and women or affect their lives except in an indirect way (see the stories of Pauline Massey and J. P. Ross).

In that great world-wide flu epidemic, over 550,000 died in the United States alone. In Tennessee, five hundred ten died in Memphis and three hundred fifty-five succumbed in Nashville. The death rate from what was called the Spanish Influenza was as high as ten per one thousand population in the state.

Pauline Massey said that in Harriman "there was a scarcity of caskets" for those who died from the effects of the flu.

Yet, none of these centenarians mentioned that they were afflicted with it.

While these men and women would be termed "strong-willed" individuals, they would also fall into the category of having a *B* type personality rather than an *A*. They were not afraid to stand up for their rights, but they were not the "rat race" leaders of the economic society. They were more followers than leaders. However, in their own fields they could be considered outstanding examples of perseverance, resourcefulness, integrity, and ability.

William Jarnagin had the oldest continuous Ford dealership in the country. John Humphreys was principal at the same school for thirty years.

The men who went to war were not the generals and admirals, but the privates and shipmates. They didn't seek acclaim and notoriety in war or in their daily lives. They did their jobs well but not as competitors with any other person.

As Mary Conley did when she insisted to her husband that she wanted to find her birth mother, they didn't mind occasionally putting a foot down and insisting on things being done their way.

In this group, you won't find those who sought high political office or climbed the corporate ladder to the top, but you will find those who took pride in whatever job they had and enjoyed doing it.

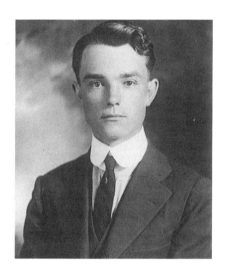 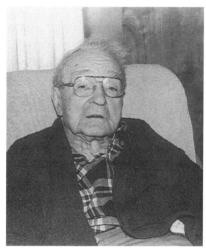

John S. Humphreys
Washington County—January 23, 1896

J ohn S. Humphreys was born three days after comedian and entertainer George Burns. Mr. Burns was ailing the day of his 100th birthday, but John S. Humphreys attended a large party in honor of his 100th birthday on January 21, 1996, just two days before his actual birthday.

Born the first of four children to Isaac Humphreys and Tima Sherfey Humphreys in their ancestral home in Johnson City, he spent his entire working life in education. From 1916 until his retirement in 1965, Mr. Humphreys served as principal at six schools in East Tennessee and as superintendent of Crockett County schools from 1926-29.

After his "retirement," he was elected to three terms on

the Board of Education where he never missed a meeting.

Everyone who reaches the milestone of one hundred years deserves a party to commemorate it and the life of the person. The only 100th Birthday Party I attended in researching the material for this book was that of John S. Humphreys. It was done up right.

Fittingly, the celebration was held in a school building (Dogwood Elementary) in South Knoxville just across the street from the honoree's home. Cars filled the parking lot, and people began arriving an hour before the scheduled time. Banners and streamers had been strung, tables set up and heaped with refreshments, and a lectern placed where notables would speak about the life of John Humphreys.

Mainly they were students. Most of them were from graduating classes of Rule High School in Knoxville where Mr. Humphreys had been principal the longest—from 1935 until 1965.

They put on name tags with the years indicating their classes. It was as much a reunion for these students as a birthday party for Mr. Humphreys. They turned out by the hundreds to honor a man who had given his life to education. He had followed in his father's footsteps, and his son and daughter followed him. His son, Jack B. Humphreys, became a professor in the Department of Civil Engineering at the University of Tennessee, and his daughter, Helen E. Knight, taught in the Nashville schools.

Those who spoke at the gathering included the Superintendent of Knox County Schools, Allen Morgan, Knox County Executive Tommy Schumpert, Mayor Victor Ashe, and Congressman Jimmy Duncan. Congressman Duncan's father, John J. Duncan, was into his first term in Congress when Mr. Humphreys retired as principal of Rule High School in 1965.

After the speeches and the presentation of a cake, plaques, and other honorary certificates, people stood in line for two hours to shake the hand of the man who had meant so much to them and to their education.

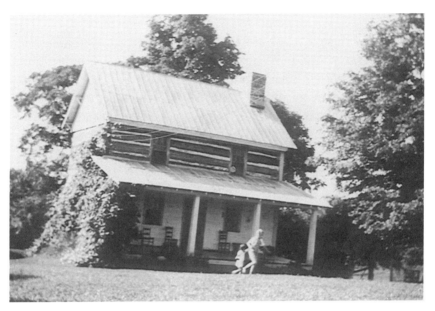

John Humphreys' birthplace was built in 1793.

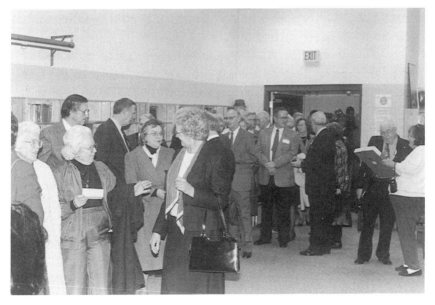

Part of the crowd at John Humphreys' 100th Birthday Party.

T he house I was born in was built in North Carolina, but I was born in Washington County, Tennessee." John Humphreys stated the little riddle to me. The house had never moved. It was built in 1793 when the territory was still part of North Carolina. Tennessee became a state in 1796, and John Humphreys was born in the two-story log home in 1896.

He was the only one I could connect to a house that was built at a time before there was a Tennessee. The house contained a great deal of Humphreys family history. His mother was born and died in the same room of the house, and now, over two hundred years after being built, it was home to a nephew who lived there and carried on the tradition.

Born four and a half miles north of Johnson City on the farm on Knob Creek, Mr. Humphreys grew up on the hundred and ten acre farm. His father later added more acreage and chores for the youngster. He remembered they raised cattle, pigs, horses, wheat, and corn. Coal oil, salt, and sugar were a few of the staples that required a trip to the store. Otherwise, the farm was self-sufficient.

As a youngster, he walked to where the *Daniel Boone* tree was in Washington County. It was reputed to be the tree on which Boone had killed a bear. "Yeah, I saw it several times. It had the carving on it. It said Boone had killed a bear on the tree and had the year carved into it."

Education was always important in the family. John attended Boone's Creek High School and then went on to East Tennessee Normal School (now East Tennessee State University). There he ran the school book store and post office to earn enough money to continue going.

"They paid me about what the food costs were at the cafeteria."

Before he graduated he was already teaching at nearby Columbia Institute at Gravel Hill. There he helped to oversee about twenty students in a two-room building. The pay was about $45 per month.

"Back then you didn't have to have a college degree to teach. If you could read and write, you could get a teaching job. Later there was a girl who had only gone through the seventh grade who was a teacher at a school where I taught."

John's father, Isaac, taught for twenty-one years. His last year was his son's first year of teaching.

From the little school in Washington County, John moved to Campbell County and became the principal of Demory Elementary just a few miles from Lafollette.

It was in Campbell County that he rode in his first car. "A friend of mine bought a car. We went to Lafollette to get it. There were three of us, maybe more. My friend never had driven a car before he bought one. So it was a little wild going back toward Demory.

"We stopped at a spring to get a drink of water. When my friend got back into the car and started up, he drove straight over the bank and into the spring. We spent a while getting the car back out. Word got back to Demory that we had been drinking and drove into the creek, but fact is, he just couldn't drive."

Some of Mr. Humphreys' fondest early memories are from his years at Demory. He was there during the time of World War I and the great influenza epidemic. The war was going on and the school didn't even have a flag. He and the students finally rounded up a flag, but they still didn't have a flagpole.

Metal was scarce and was needed for the war effort. Principal Humphreys resorted to an East Tennessee resource. The chestnut tree blight had already hit many of the great trees of the area.

"We took a dead chestnut tree, cut it down, and painted it red, white, and blue. We were finally able to get it into a hole in front of the school house. We had one fine flagpole."

Mr. Humphreys taught and principaled at other schools across the state until settling in Knoxville in 1929. "Every school I was principal at, I also taught at."

The school term was a lot shorter when he was in Campbell County. Some schools went five months and some seven. "Some students would get out of their five-month term and then come to my school at Demory for the other two months."

School was turned out for reasons we don't think about today.

"Molasses. We had to turn school out at molasses making time in the fall. The students had to go home and help their families with the chores and making molasses."

When he came to Knoxville to be principal at Lonsdale Elementary, Mr. Humphreys was able to further his own education by attending the University of Tennessee. There he obtained his bachelor's and master's degrees during the 1930s.

At Rule, which was soon to be Rule High, Mr. Humphreys settled into his last job in education—for thirty years.

It was hundreds of these students who came back to share with Mr. Humphreys, their teacher, principal, and friend, on the celebration of his attaining one hundred years of age.

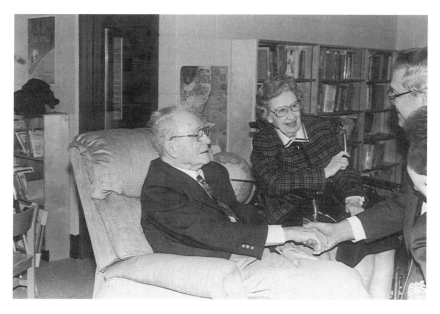

Mr. Humphreys and wife, Florence, greet well-wishers.

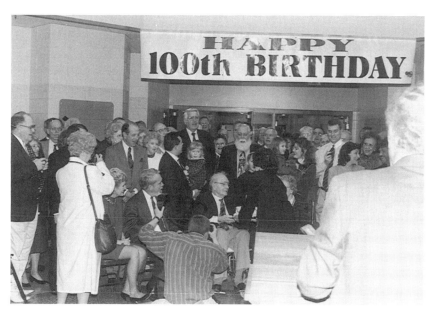

Family and friends gather at Knoxville's Dogwood Elementary

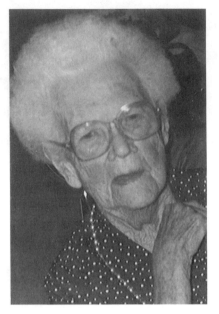

Mary Cartwright Abston Conley
Putnam County—December 23, 1890

E very morning before breakfast, my daddy would get a tall stemmed glass, fill it with whiskey, sugar, and water, and pass it around the table for everybody to have a swallow. He said it kept away illness. It was the way we started every day." That was the only drinking of alcoholic beverages Mary Conley said she did during her life.

I talked with Mary at her room in the Johnson Health Care Center in Harriman, Tennessee, just ten days after she turned 105. Something shooed illness and the doctors away from this vigorous lady who had kept her own apartment until she was 102.

The sugary whiskey wasn't her earliest memory. She squinted her eyes and thought back to when she was four years old.

"Times were hard. My mother had me and two little brothers. I remember her trying to find food for us. It was a late spring day. The only thing she could find was an apple tree with a few small apples that she put in a bucket, and we walked home." They lived in rural Putnam County. Mary doesn't remember her real father.

"A couple who lived a ways down the road came along and saw that my mother was having a hard time. They asked to take me. My mother told them, 'No.' Then they asked just to keep me overnight so that they could get me a good meal.

"I went with them. The next thing I know they had gone to court and adopted me. I didn't see my real mother again until after I was married." Her birth mother was Rosetta Cartwright.

Mary is the only centenarian in this book who was adopted. It wasn't that unusual when times were hard for uncles, aunts, or cousins to take in their kinfolk and adopt the young children. But as far as Mary remembers, Thomas and Zillie Abston were not blood-relatives of hers. They adopted her because they thought they could not have children after being married for nine years. After the adoption, her new parents had children of their own.

The "Good Ole Days" weren't the way she recalled her new relationship. "If slaves had to work any harder than I had to work, I wouldn't believe it.

"One day there was snow on the ground, and my father decided it would be a good time for me to cut the weeds and briars that had grown up around the buildings. He said I could make a little fire out of kindling and burn the weeds and briars in that too. Snow was up to my shoes. Finally, my mother saw me out there working and told me to get back into the house. It wasn't suitable weather to be doing that kind of work outside.

"My father got mad about it and rode away on the mule. We didn't see him for a day."

I wondered how her birthday coming so near Christmas affected her celebrations during her younger years. "We didn't celebrate Christmas. If it was working weather, we worked."

Mary either had or developed a strong-willed character trait. She was tough in body and mind.

"I went to the ninth grade at Pleasant Hill Academy but had to drop out because of family problems. I was out of school for about five years when I turned twenty.

"I sat down and wrote the professor at the school and asked him if I could come back to school. He wrote me back and said he'd be delighted to have me back.

"My mother got the letter and didn't want me to go. But I went anyway. I was of age. I remember the professor having somebody from the school come to my house. There were two white horses pulling a buggy. I got my bag and walked to the buggy.

"There were two dormitories for girls and one for boys at the school."

Mary didn't get to finish her education. Illness of a brother brought her back home and then to a cousin's to live.

She married the next year, 1913.

A year or so after she married, Mary told her husband that she wanted to go and see her birth mother, Rosetta Cartwright.

"He told me he'd take me. After several months passed, he hadn't, and I asked him again. He told me he wasn't going to and to forget about it.

"I packed my bag and took out on foot to find my mother. I went through woods, walked through creeks, and over ridges, but I finally got there. I stayed six weeks before I went back to my husband. When I wanted to do anything, I did it!"

Mary and her husband had ten children. Four of them died at or near birth. They had a little farm, but her husband mainly worked in the coal mines. He was injured in a rock fall in the mine and never fully recovered. He died in 1960.

Since then, Mary Conley lived in Ohio with a child for twelve years and then moved back to Tennessee. Here she has lived near another child and lived with her son-in-law after a daughter's death. In her nineties, she moved into a residential apartment complex for the elderly.

"I really liked that. I had my own bedroom, a living room, a bathroom and a kitchen. We'd go and buy groceries, and I cooked. I was on the third floor, and my window faced the Emory River. In the evening, I could sit near the window and watch the boats on the water."

Mary was always a healthy, hearty, robust, and independent woman.

"I never even saw a doctor until after I was married. I birthed all of my children at home without a doctor."

She eats about anything she wants but doesn't care much for the food at the facility where she lives now. She pieces quilts together, reads large print books, sews some, and watches television.

"I can look out the window here, but I feel like I'm down in a hole too much to see anything."

There were still cakes, cookies, and candy around from her birthday party two weeks before. "I never did eat much sweets. Take some if you want," she offered.

Mary Cartwright Abston Conley—she always gave more than she took.

Two Missing

A s I did research and interviews for this book, I often missed opportunities to talk with some who had passed 100 because I was too late. They had died before I found time to visit them.

Then there were two women, one 101 and the other 105, whom I visited but who did not want their stories told. What was the reason? I sat and talked with each for at least a half hour, but they would never consent to "going on the record" for purposes of this book. They would not talk about the past except in brief answers about parents or such.

Were they hiding deep, dark secrets? No. I finally concluded that they didn't want any notoriety about them because of their age. They would talk about the present much more freely than the past.

One said, "People just look at me as a curiosity piece because I'm over a hundred." She went on to talk about baseball and basketball and the latest polls in *USA Today*. She looked more like seventy than one hundred.

Again, these two demonstrated the strong-willed characteristic that I found in most of these centenarians.

Everyone has a right to privacy, to be left alone, and not be bothered. In our everyday living, we need to be careful as to how we treat our elderly. We must remember they are just like us—only older. They are not curiosity pieces to be gawked at. They shouldn't be met with everyone asking how old they are, and then receive an astonished look which to them could mean, "You should be dead."

About twenty years ago, I was at a branch bank opening where the master of ceremonies was introducing all the dignitaries including the bank's oldest customer.

"Mr. Smith is here today," the bright young man said. "He is one hundred and one years old. And he's still living. Would you please stand, Mr. Smith?"

The old man was much kinder than I would have been. He stood and waved to the crowd instead of saying, "If I wasn't living, I wouldn't be here."

In our families and in our communities, the elderly, and especially those who reach a hundred or more years, generally want to be treated the same as we would treat people of half their age—with respect and consideration.

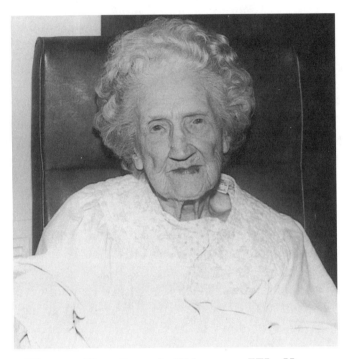

Tom Garland Kinser Wallace
Monroe County—February 25, 1895

I n the year of Tennessee's Bicentennial, Tom Wallace has more than most to celebrate. She turned 101, and her ancestor, Colonel Samuel Wear, was one of the original signers of Tennessee's constitution at the formation of the state. Half as old as the state, she was born one year before the centennial of the signing of the historical document.

Born between Vonore and Madisonville, Tom moved with her parents to Knoxville when she was ten years old. They lived downtown near the Southern Railway depot. Her mother ran a boarding house for some of the railroaders, and that was where Tom met her husband-to-be.

"At the time, I was sort of going with another young

man who lived there. I wasn't too crazy about him. So, one evening I was sitting in the swing on the porch, and my boyfriend had stepped out for a while. Mr. (W. G.) Wallace came over and said he would like to vie for my affections. I said, 'That's fine with me.'

"We were married when I was about sixteen. We went on the train to New York on our honeymoon. We stopped in Bristol and Washington.

"After a bit in New York, I wanted to see the sights. My husband said he didn't want to go. I just took off. Left him at the hotel, and I saw the sights. I walked over one of those big bridges. I walked up into the Statue of Liberty. Had a big time."

Tom was the oldest of three sisters and learned to take charge early.

She was named Tom Garland because they were both family names and her grandmother insisted to her mother that she name her first heir with the family names.

"Did it bother you, or did the other children tease you about being named Tom?" I asked.

"No," she said. "It didn't bother me."

Neither her husband nor she ever owned an automobile.

"How did you get around?"

"My husband worked for the railroad. He started as the telegraph operator. We road the train. He got passes. We went to Chicago and Texas. Around town, I would ride the electric street cars and later the buses. I walked a lot. Never had a car."

"Did you register to vote in 1920?"

"You bet I did. And I always voted. I'm a Democrat."

She and her husband had no children. Tom began to work at Watson's in downtown Knoxville. "I worked in piece goods for years and years. It was back when they had the Market House there near Watson's. You could walk through the Market House and smell the fish from one end to the other. The farmers would sell their vegetables and fruits beside the building."

Mrs. Wallace said she liked almost all foods. When she was a youngster and lived in Monroe County, she would get in trouble from time to time when she tried to rob her grandmother Harvey's pie safe. "Oh, yeah, she had to spank me to keep me away from those pies."

Later, after she married, her mother continued to live with her, and they made fried pies together. Her favorite though is still an egg custard pie.

It was a week after Valentine's Day and the day after Presidents' Day when I talked with Mrs. Wallace. She was living at the Shannondale Retirement Center in west Knoxville.

"Do you have a favorite President?" I asked.

She had to think for a minute. "Well, it would have to be a Democrat. Roosevelt, I guess. Franklin Roosevelt. They have his picture and some of the other Presidents up out in the lobby."

She had never been hospitalized or operated on until she had a burn on her legs shortly before going to Shannondale. She was a charter member of Central United Methodist Church and her Sunday School room has been named in her honor. She is religious and entertains the staff at Shannondale with her singing.

Mrs. Wallace's husband died in 1958. She didn't remarry and continued to keep her residence at her house until just a few years before I saw her. "I guess I'll stay here the rest of my life. I get good care here."

It was at this point that a nurse stepped into the room. "Are you going to be much longer?" she asked.

"Not much," I said.

"Well, I don't mean to rush you, but Mrs. Wallace's boyfriend is down the hall crying. He saw her come into her room with you and thought she had a new boyfriend."

Mrs. Wallace's eyes lighted up. I knew it was time for the interview to be over and closed up my pad. She got to her feet, and with the help of a walker, started down the hallway to the area where her friend waited. Her pace was faster than when she walked into the room with me.

When I passed by, she had found her friend. They sat side by side, holding hands. The nurses were changing shifts. Some stopped, smiled, and applauded the love and caring.

Tom Garland Wallace's mother was Elizabeth Lucretia Harvey Kinser, b. 5-26-1871, d. 2-5-1944. Her father was L. L. Kinser. On her mother's side, her grandparents were Newton Lafayette Harvey, b. 11-16-1843, d. 4-27-1915; and Mary Jane Smith Harvey, b. 11-10-1844, d. 5-20-1932; great-grandparents Thomas G. Harvey, b. 1815, d. 1895, and Lucretia Adeline Wear (grand-daughter of Colonel Samuel Wear) b.1822, d. 1874.

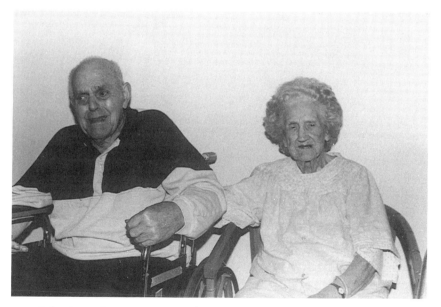

Mrs. Tom Garland Wallace shares a quiet moment with her friend.

Enjoy It!

I took pleasure when I could. I acted clearly and morally and without regret. I'm very lucky." Those are the words of the world's oldest (as I write this in February 1996) woman, Jeanne Calment, 121, of France.

The world's oldest man, Chris Mortenson, 113, of San Rafael, California, told a *Parade* magazine correspondent, "I was always a very independent kind of man. That helped me reach 113."

Summed up in these two statements of ordinary people who lived what we consider extremely long lives are the secrets to longevity and productivity.

Mr. Mortenson said what we found to be true among these Tennessee centenarians—strong-willed independence is a touch stone. In both men and women, independence was either acquired or inherited. Reread these mini-biographies and you will see again and again the story of self-reliance and an independent spirit.

Whether she meant that she was *very lucky* to live to 120 or *very lucky* to have such a good life of however many years, Jeanne Calment was right on both counts.

Luck, good fortune, providence, or whatever also played a role in the lives of these centenarians. War didn't kill them. They bypassed airplane crashes. They were not crippled by other accidents. They had food, clothing, and shelter enough to survive at all times. So, we would have to say that good fortune may be just as important as good genes in survival to the century mark.

"I acted clearly and morally," Ms. Calment said. Again these are two of the characteristics of the Tennessee centenarians. Decision making was done after reflection and with a regard for others and themselves. There was a deep religiosity among the great majority. They were bright people, whether college educated or not. They read, they wrote, they built, they sold, they played musical instruments, they rode horses (and later they drove cars), they voted, they cared for their families, and they cared for themselves.

The Bible teaches that the second greatest commandment is to "love thy neighbor as thyself." Lev. 19:18 and Mark 12:31. These centenarians seemed to have followed that instruction for the most part. They loved those they were around, and they loved *themselves.* In all that they did, they practiced moderation and balance.

Without regret. There's no turning the clock back. There's no undoing things that were done wrong or half-done. If they were asked, most all of these centenarians could think of an example of where they could have done better in a situation or with a problem. But, as Ms. Calment said, when it was done, they went on—*without regret.* Not looking back, but rather looking forward, is another key to a long, productive, and enjoyable life.

A sense of place, a sense of family, putting grief in its place, developing socialization skills, and being of medium build all appeared important qualities that these centenarians shared. But none is more important than what Jeanne Calment, the world's oldest woman, said: *"I took pleasure when I could."*

Traveling through life, all of these centenarians seemed to have *enjoyed it*—and even better, they all seemed still to be enjoying it at 100!

There are those who drag through life. They will enjoy things when they **retire.** They will enjoy things when the **children grow up.** They will enjoy things when they get a bigger car, a better house, their promotion, or win the lottery.

These centenarians teach us to enjoy it as we go.

Enjoyment to them was more than a giddy happiness, frivolity, or some celebratory excess. They found enjoyment in helping to bring lights to Rutledge, in making a quilt for a young man, in contributing to their communities, states, nation, and families.

The *pursuit of happiness* they read about in the Declaration of Independence was not a license for lascivious living, but instead their pursuit of happiness was a constructive citizenship.

They found little joys in everyday living. Teaching a student, tending the garden, making a quilt, caring for orphaned nephews and nieces, surveying for a new road, playing the violin or the piano, or learning a new language.

Enjoyment was wrapped up in family, friends, and home—not wild parties.

As America prepares for the new century and the new millenium, the troubling spectre of drug use permeates our society. A lesson from these centenarians is understated. They found enjoyment from *within* and not from *without* in the use of alcohol or drugs to excess.

There is a generation of Americans today seeking enjoyment through excitement and "highs" in drug use. Unfortunately, this book will be lost on most of them. They either don't expect to live to 100 or wouldn't want to if they had to live such "boring" lives. Few of them read anything and certainly not a book about old folks.

It was the Apostle Paul who said, "For I have learned, in whatsoever state I am, therewith to be content.

"I know how to be abased, and I know how to abound: everywhere and in all things I am instructed both to be full and to be hungry, both to abound and to suffer need.

"I can do all things through Christ which strengtheneth me." (Phil. 4: 11-13)

Contentment and enjoyment walk hand in hand—like an elderly couple strolling down a beach or along a country lane. It is difficult to see the one without the other.

In Conclusion

Whether we reach a hundred years of age or not, the quality of life and enjoyment can be increased with careful consideration of the lives of these centenarians and others you may know who have found where happiness lies.

Those who live beyond their 80s appear to have a good quality of life, often right up to the end. Very few are hospitalized for any length of time. They do not require much in the way of medical care and therefore are not a burden on their families or on society. When the end comes, it usually is swift with virtually no lingering. (Many of those in this book passed from this life quickly when it was time.)

While there are about 52,000 centenarians in the United States now, it is expected that the number will swell to over 1.3 million before the *Baby Boomers* move through.

Is it too late to do anything to improve our quality of life to where we can enjoy living to a hundred if the opportunity is given? In my estimation, No! While we can't obtain a new gene pool or change the family we came from, there are simple things we can do to insure a quality life.

From these centenarians, I see a quality life as one that is focused on others and not ourselves, one that is more full of people than things, one that has meaning and direction, and one that always looks to the future and not the past. Our emphasis should be on a life that has deep satisfaction and enjoyment through concern for others and our communities. Once life becomes unenjoyable, it often ends.

As more and more Tennesseans and Americans live into their 80s, 90s, and past the 100 year barrier, what will society do with them? That, perhaps, is the biggest question.

Some societies revere their elderly as being wise with so many years of experiences held within them. For some time, we have been different in this country. At 65, or perhaps 70, senior citizens are encouraged to retire, to quit their vocations, to shrivel up and go away. We are attuned to the young, the energetic, the enthusiastic, and we imply that those over 70 cannot continue to have these attributes.

One challenge for America as we enter a new century is to find new and rewarding opportunities for our elderly. Their wealth of knowledge and experience could well be put to good uses if we think ahead. And if we do that, it will benefit our communities, states, and nation. It will also give to those older Americans a sense of usefulness and make their latter years more enjoyable and fulfilling.

While many more people will be living to a hundred, very few reach 110. The oldest ones that I interviewed for this book were 105. Those who study such things tell us that the life *span* of humans is about 120—meaning that is about the limit of humans' ability to live. Life *expectancy,* on the other hand, is the average number of years that we can expect to live. In the United States, that is now in the high seventies.

The hundred years just past saw more changes than any century in history. These men and women were witnesses to a century like no other. They are to be honored and commended. The changes of the next century offer a challenge to us. May we meet them with the same equanimity.

May all your years, however many they may be, be filled with joy!

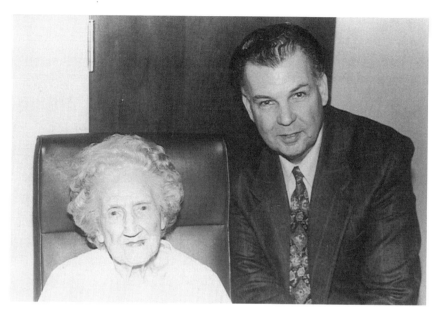

Tom Garland Wallace (left) with author Chris Cawood.

About the Author

Chris Cawood lives in Kingston, Tennessee, where he practices law and writes. He is a 1970 graduate of the University of Tennessee College of Law. He is a member of the 1965 Class of Karns High School in Knox County.

From 1974-78, he was a member of the Tennessee General Assembly, representing parts of Roane, Anderson, Morgan, and Campbell Counties.

He is married to the former Sara Fowler of Kimball, Tennessee, and they have two children, Shannon and Suzanne, and a daughter-in-law Ruthie.

Order other books by Chris Cawood

For an autographed copy of *How To Live To 100*, send $10 (includes postage and any applicable tax) to Magnolia Hill Press, P.O. Box 124, Kingston, Tennessee 37763.

Tennessee's Coal Creek War—a historical novel of an 1890s love story set against the backdrop of a coal miners' rebellion in East Tennessee. Softcover $12.

The Legacy of The Swamp Rat—The story of the Tennessee vs. Alabama football series and the Volunteer quarterbacks who just said *NO* to Alabama. Hardback—$10.

1998: The Year of The Beast—a political, murder mystery set in New Orleans, Washington, Kentucky, and Tennessee. Softcover, 312 pages, $12.

Phone 1-800-946-1967 to place VISA or Mastercard orders.